Dr Sebi Cookbook

More Than 150 Recipes to Lose Weight and Improve Your Life with first courses, Main courses, Side Dishes and Delicious Smoothies Based on Dr Sebi's Alkaline Diet

Moyra Eimhir Mcneal

material may be claimed by the holder of this copyright.

The data, depictions, events, descriptions, and all other information forthwith are considered to be true, fair, and accurate unless the work is expressly described as a work of fiction. Regardless of the nature of this work, the Publisher is exempt from any responsibility for actions taken by the reader in conjunction with this work. The Publisher acknowledges that the reader acts of their own accord and releases the author and Publisher of any responsibility for the observance of tips, advice, counsel, strategies, and techniques that may be offered in this volume.

Dr SEBI COOKBOOK

Table of Contents

Introduction

Congratulations on purchasing *Dr Sebi Smoothie,* and thank you for doing so.
The recipes included within this book are plant-based and follow the rules of the Dr. Sebi Alkaline Diet.

Dr. Sebi is a naturalist, pathologist, biochemist, herbalist who studied and personally observed herbs in North and South America, the Caribbean, and Africa. He developed a unique approach to healing the human body using herbs firmly rooted in over 30 years of experience. Dr. Sebi created a line of natural vegetable cell food compounds used for inter-cellular cleansing and cellular revitalization.

Before we begin, I want to give a brief disclaimer: This book is not intended to replace medical advice. It is not responsible for the actions or the results of the reader. Please seek out the advice of a doctor before starting any health program. The author is not a medical doctor. This book's information is meant only to supplement your health decisions and actions, not dictate them. The nuances of inflammation are still being discovered as this book is being written. Please enjoy the information provided but also be wise in consuming it.

Throughout the book, you will see burro bananas. They resemble the cavendish variety but are shorter and more square in shape with dark green peels that deepen to deep yellow with black spots when matured. They possess a creamy yellow or white flesh. They have a lemon-banana flavor when mature and are slightly firmer toward the center.

You will also see several products to prepare some of Dr. Sebi's recipes. These are what you need:

- Dr. Sebi's Nerve/Stress Relief Herbal Tea
- Dr. Sebi's Stomach Relief Herbal Tea
- Dr. Sebi's Immune Support Herbal Tea

You will also need to have soft-jelly coconut milk. Youtube provides a video:
https://www.youtube.com/watch?v=1kNk8zP83w
s

Sea Moss Gel is another product used with Dr. Sebi's recipes. Here is how to make it:

Total Time Required: 10 minutes
Yields Provided: 32 tablespoons

Ingredients Needed:

- Dried whole sea moss (1 cup - packed)
- Spring water (1-2 cups)

Instructions:

Prepare The Sea Moss

1. Remove the sea moss from its package. Thoroughly rinse your seaweed with filtered or spring water - *not* tap water.
2. Fill a container with water. Add the sea moss in and soak in spring or filtered water for four to eight hours or overnight.

Prepare the Sea Moss Gel

1. Once it's soaked, drain the liquid from the bowl.
2. Pour in more fresh spring water with the moss into a high-speed blender. Pulse it for one to two minutes until it's completely smooth.
3. Pour the mixture into a glass jar and securely close with a lid.
4. Pop it into the fridge until it creates a gel.
5. You can use it in homemade jams, raw vegan desserts, vegan bread, soups, and smoothies.
6. The sea moss gel will remain safe when stored in the fridge for three to four weeks and in the freezer for two to three months.

Now, let's begin!

Chapter 1
<u>Breakfast Favorites</u>

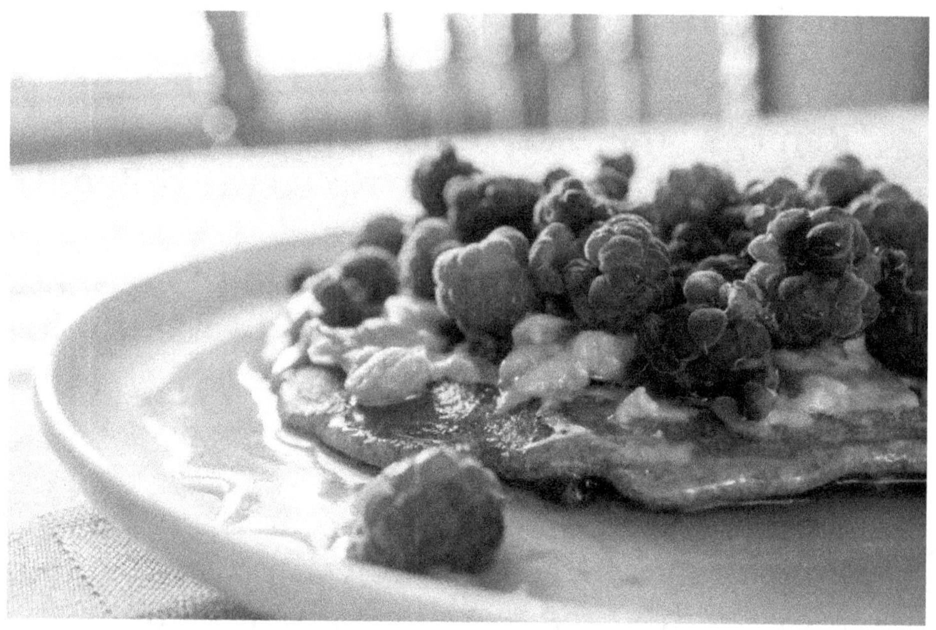

Fixings to Get Started

<u>Brazil Nut Cheese</u>

Total Time Required: 5 minutes + soak time (2 hours)

Yields Provided: 6 cups

Ingredients Needed:
- Soaked Brazil nuts* (1 lb./450 g)
- Lime juice (half of 1 lime)

- Sea salt (2 tsp.)
- Cayenne (.5 tsp.)
- Onion powder (1 tsp.)
- Hemp milk (1.5 cups)
- Spring Water (1.5 cups)
- Grapeseed oil (2 tsp.)
- Food processor or blender also needed

Instructions:

1. It is recommended to soak the nuts overnight, but two hours will suffice.
2. Toss all of the fixings into the blender (minus the water).
3. Slowly begin by adding ½ cup of water to combine the fixings (2 min.).
4. Continue adding water (½ cup), blending until the preferred texture is attained.

Dr. Sebi Inspired Whipped Cream

Total Time Required: 15-20 minutes
Yields Provided: Approx. 1 cup

Ingredients Needed:
- Aquafaba (1 cup)
- Agave (.25 cup)
- Stand/Hand mixer

Instructions:

1. Measure and add the agave and aquafaba into a big mixing container. Blend it using the high-speed setting.
2. Prep times will vary; the stand mixer (5 min.) and the hand mixer (10-15 min.).
3. It's ready for use.
4. Note: After use, always place it back into the fridge. As time passes, the whipped cream will revert back to aquafaba. All you need to do is whip it again to revive it back to whipped cream.

Fresh Tamarind Water
Total Time Required: 25 minutes

Ingredients Needed:
- Tamarind pulp (3.5 oz./100 g)
- Boiling spring water (20 fl oz./600 ml)
- Fresh spring water (2.1 quarts/2 liters)
- Date sugar/Agave syrup

Instructions:

1. Pour boiling water over the tamarind pulp, and set it aside to soak (20 min.).
2. Break the pulp apart. Strain the mixture into a mixing dish using a sieve, pressing as much pulp through as possible using a spoon.
3. Scrape any tamarind puree from the underside of the sieve into the mixing container. Rinse the liquids using a liter of fresh spring water.
4. Sweeten with agave syrup or date sugar to taste.

All-Natural Tamarind Paste

Ingredients Needed:
- Natural tamarind (8.8 oz./250 g)
- Springwater (3 cups)
- *A high-speed blender is needed.

Instructions:

1. Clean the tamarind, checking for any seeds, skin, or unwanted particles, and discard them.
2. Warm two cups of water to soak the tamarind (45 min. to 1 hr.)
3. Once the tamarind is softened, blend it until it's creamy.
4. Pass the resulting mixture through a sifter, discarding any stones, seeds, or other debris.
5. Boil the pulp for five minutes using the medium-temperature setting.
6. Once the paste is completely cooled, store in airtight containers.

Hemp Milk

Total Time Required: 5 minutes + chilling time (2 hrs.)
Yields Provided: 2 cups

Ingredients Needed:
- Hemp seeds (2 tbsp.)
- Spring water (2 cups)
- Agave (2 tbsp.)
- Sea salt (.125 tsp./a pinch)
- Optional: Strawberries (1 cup)

Instructions:

1. Pour each of the fixings, except the fruit, into a blender.
2. Blend for two minutes.
3. Add fruit to the milk and blend for ½ minute.
4. Store milk in the fridge for one to two hours or until it's chilled as desired.

Quinoa Milk

Total Time Required: 10 minutes
Yields Provided: 4

Ingredients Needed:
- Cooked white quinoa (1 cup)
- Spring water (3 cups)
- Dates (6-8)
- Cloves (1 pinch/optional)
- Sea salt (1 pinch/optional)
- Milk bag/Cheesecloth

Instructions:

1. Toss all of the fixings into a blender. Pulse them for 45-60 seconds.
2. Strain and store it safely in the fridge for three to four days.

Walnut Milk

Total Time Required: 5 minutes
Yields Provided: 12 @ .25 cup each

Ingredients Needed:
- Walnuts (1 cup)
- Filtered watered (3.5 cups)
- Cinnamon (.25 tsp.)

Instructions:

1. There are two options for making this recipe.
2. If you're in a hurry, boil the walnuts for ten minutes to soften them. Option two is to soak them overnight for at least eight hours.
3. Strain/ rinse soaked or boiled walnuts.
4. Toss the strained walnuts in a blender. Add filtered water and cinnamon.
5. Blend on high for one minute until smooth.
6. Strain the mixture through a nut milk bag (there should be minimal pulp with walnuts).
7. Pour it into a Mason jar and pop it in the fridge to enjoy for up to four days.

Pancakes

Alkaline Delicious Breakfast Patties

Total Time Required: 10-15 minutes
Yields Provided: 6 patties

Ingredients Needed:
- Spelt flour (.5 cup)
- Garbanzo bean flour (.5 cup)
- Thyme (.5 tsp.)
- Approved herb of choice (.5 tsp.)
- Sage (1 tsp.)
- Ground clove (1 pinch)
- Crushed red pepper (.5 tsp.)
- Sea salt (.5 tsp.)
- Cayenne (1 pinch)
- Spring water (.5 cup)
- Grapeseed oil (1 tbsp.)

Instructions:

1. Toss and thoroughly mix the fixings in a mixing container till it becomes pasty.
2. Pour a bit of oil into a frying pan. Warm it using the med-high temperature setting.
3. Add the patty batter to the skillet, flipping them every three minutes until done.

Dr. Sebi's Owl Blueberry Pancakes

Total Time Required: 20 minutes
Yields Provided: varies

Ingredients Needed:
- Homemade walnut milk (1.25 cups)
- Spelt - Amaranth or Kamut flour (1.5 cups)
- Date sugar (3 tbsp.)
- Sea salt (1 pinch)
- Grapeseed oil (2 tbsp.)
- Blueberries (.33 cup)
- To Serve: Fruit & agave syrup

Instructions:

1. Preheat a skillet/griddle to 350° Fahrenheit/177° Celsius or the medium-temperature setting.
2. Brush the pan using a spritz of grapeseed oil.
3. Whisk the flour and sugar until it's smooth.
4. Pour the oil and milk into the flour-date sugar mixture.
5. Briskly beat until most of the flour is incorporated.
6. Fold in the blueberries using a spatula to maintain lumps. *Don't overmix.*

7. Add 0.25 to 0.33 cup portions of the batter into the skillet. Gently spread it out using a spoon to reach the desired shape.
8. Cook until the bottom is golden and the edges are slightly cooked (2-3 min.).
9. Flip and continue to cook until that side is golden as well (1-2 min.).
10. Serve with agave syrup and extra fruit to make the "owl" shapes.

5-Ingredient Pancakes

Total Time Required: 20-25 minutes
Yields Provided: 12 pancakes

Ingredients Needed:
- Raw sesame "tahini" butter (.25 cup)
- Walnut milk (1 cup)
- Agave syrup (6 tbsp.)
- Kamut flour (1 cup)
- Grapeseed oil (1 tbsp.)

Instructions:

1. Whisk the butter with agave syrup and milk in a mixing container.
2. Fold in the Kamut flour, stirring until it's thoroughly combined.
3. Warm a skillet using the medium-temperature setting.
4. Once it's hot, add a drizzle of oil. Remove any excess fat with a paper towel.
5. Scoop the batter (2 tbsp.) into the pan. Wait for the bubbles - about one minute.
6. Flip the pancakes. Wait roughly half a minute before transferring them onto a plate.
7. Repeat until you've finished the batter and have a stack of pancakes.
8. Serve with fresh fruit and a bit of agave syrup.

Green Pancakes

Total Time Required: 15 minutes
Yields Provided: 3 large/6 small cakes

Ingredients Needed:

- Chickpea flour (.5 cup)
- Sea salt (.5 tsp.)
- Fresh spring water (.5 cup)
- Blueberries (.25 cup)
- Burro banana (1)
- Agave syrup (1 tbsp.)
- Amaranth greens (1 handful)
- Nut butter of choice - adds more protein (homemade tahini/walnut/Brazil nut (1 tbsp.)

Instructions:

1. Toss each of the fixings into a blender. Mix until smooth. Use caution not to add too much water, or they will not be as fluffy.
2. Allow the batter to sit for five to ten minutes.
3. Warm a skillet over a med-high temperature setting.
4. Scoop the batter into the pan to form six small pancakes, three large or four to five medium ones.

5. Cook the pancakes until there are some bubbles in the batter. The edges should be browning.
6. Turn them over and continue cooking (2-3 min.).
7. Decorate and serve with a few bananas, blueberries, and agave syrup.

Zucchini Bread Pancakes

Total Time Required: 20 minutes
Yields Provided: 12-14 - varies.

Ingredients Needed:
- Spelt or Kamut flour (2 cups)
- Date sugar (2 tbsp.)
- Mashed burro banana (.25 cup)
- Finely shredded zucchini (1 cup)
- Homemade walnut milk (2 cups)
- Chopped walnuts (.5 cup)
- Grapeseed oil (1 tbsp.)

Instructions:

1. Prepare a big mixing container to whisk the flour with the date sugar.
2. Pour in the milk and mashed burro banana. Stir until just combined.
3. Shred and mix in walnuts and shredded zucchini.
4. Warm the oil in a griddle/skillet using a med-high temperature setting.
5. Pour the batter onto the griddle to cook your pancakes (4-5 min. per side).
6. Serve with agave syrup.

Other Treats

"Alkaline" Blackberry Breakfast Bars

Total Time Required: 30 minutes
Yields Provided: 8

Ingredients Needed:
- Baby bananas (4) or Burro bananas (3)
- Grapeseed oil (.5 cup)
- Agave nectar (.25 cup)
- Quinoa flakes (2 cups)
- Sea salt (.25 tsp.)
- Spelt flour (1 cup)
- Alkaline Blackberry Jam - see below for recipe**(1 cup)

Instructions:

1. Set the oven temperature setting to 350° Fahrenheit/177° Celsius.
2. Mash the bananas in a big mixing container.
3. Add the oil and agave nectar to the bananas, mixing until incorporated.
4. Into the wet mixture, add your quinoa flakes, sea salt, and spelt flour.
5. Mix all of the ingredients to create a sticky dough when pressed between your fingers.

6. Evenly press ⅔ of the mixture into a 9 x 9-inch square parchment paper-lined pan.
7. Spread the *Blackberry Jam* (recipe below) over the top. Top it off using the remaining of your dough mixture crumbling evenly.
8. Bake for 20 minutes uncovered.
9. Once it's done, transfer it to the countertop for the bars to cool about 15 minutes before cutting.
10. These bars will last in the refrigerator for about five to six days.
11. Pop them into the freezer for a shelf life of about three months
12. These bars work with any type of fruit jam. If you are using store-bought blackberry jam, you will use less (like ½ cup) since the store-bought jam is much sweeter.

The Blackberry Jam

Total Time Required: 17 minutes
Yields Provided: 43 tablespoons

Ingredients Needed:
- Fresh blackberries (3 pkg. @ 6 oz. each)
- Agave nectar (3 tbsp.)
- Squeezed key lime juice (1 tbsp.)
- Sea moss gel (0.25 cup + 2 tbsp.)

Instructions:

1. Rinse the blackberries and toss them into a medium-size pot.
2. Heat them using the med-high temperature setting. Stir until the juices from the berries begin to disperse.
3. Use an immersion blender, potato masher, or food processor/blender to break down any remaining big pieces.
4. Mix in the agave nectar, and sea moss gel, and key lime juice. Stir until your jam starts to thicken (1-2 min.) using the med-low temperature setting. The sea moss gel will thicken the jam pretty quick.
5. Remove the pan from the hot burner to cool (15 min.).

6. Use it on toast, pancakes, waffles, or as desired!
7. If not using immediately, scoop it into a clean, sterile mason jar. Be sure the lid closes tightly. Keep the container in the fridge to enjoy for five to seven days. It will also freeze nicely for up to about two months.

Dr. Sebi's Inspired Donuts

Total Time Required: 20-25 minutes
Yields Provided: 6-12 donuts - depending on pan size

Ingredients Needed:
- Garbanzo bean/Chickpea flour (.75 cup)
- Spelt flour (.75 cup)
- Sparkling spring water (.25 cup)
- Agave (.75 cup)
- Grapeseed oil (2 tsp.)
- Sea salt (.5 tsp.)
- Sea Moss Gel (1 tsp.)
- Cloves - ground (.25 tsp.)
- Alkaline applesauce - see the recipe (.25 cup)

Instructions:

1. Add all ingredients, except the grapeseed oil, into a big mixing container and whisk until it's thoroughly incorporated.
2. Lightly brush donut pan with oil.
3. Preheat the oven to 350° Fahrenheit/177° Celsius.
4. Pour batter into donut pan about 3/4 of the way to the top.
5. Bake for 12-14 minutes.

6. Allow donuts to cool, then cut out the centers if needed, based on pan type.
7. Top off with Alkaline Frosting (below) or glaze with coconut flakes.

Dr. Sebi's Inspired Frosting

Total Time Required: 20 minutes
Yields Provided: 12 oz. frosting

Ingredients Needed:
- Creamed coconut (7 oz./200 g)
- Hemp milk (.5 cup)
- Agave (.25 cup)
- Strawberries or blueberries - Freeze-dried (.25 cup/optional)
- *Pure* vanilla extract*** (.5 tsp./optional)
- Pestle & mortar
- Stick mixer preferred - a handheld will work.

***Vanilla is *not* on "Dr. Sebi's Nutritional Guide." However, he has stated that "it's okay to add in small amounts. Be sure to use pure vanilla extract - not imitation".

Instructions:

1. Blend the creamed coconut with the agave and milk (¼ cup) until it's thoroughly mixed and creamy.
2. Crush the fruit into a powder and whip it into the frosting.

Pour in the rest of the milk or as needed to reach the preferred consistency

Dr. Sebi's Inspired Sausage Links

Total Time Required: 20-25 minutes
Yields Provided: 15-20 links

Ingredients Needed:
- Mushrooms (1 cup)
- Cooked garbanzo beans (2 cups)
- Garbanzo bean flour (.5 cup)
- Roma tomato (1)
- Oregano (1 tsp.)
- Chopped onion (.5 cup)
- Onion powder (1 tbsp.)
- Ground sage (1 tsp.)
- Sea salt (1 tsp.)
- Dill (1 tsp.)
- Ground cloves (.5 tsp.)
- Regular/sweet basil (1 tsp.)
- Cayenne powder (.5 tsp.)
- Grapeseed oil (2 tbsp./as needed)
- Food Processor

Instructions:

1. Excluding the garbanzo flour, toss all of the fixings into the processor.
2. Pulse the mixture (10 sec.).
3. Mix in the flour till it's thoroughly mixed (20 sec.).

4. Scoop the mixture into a piping bag.
5. Add oil (2 tbsp.) into a skillet using the medium-high temperature setting.
6. Work the blend into links and place in the heated pan.
7. Cook for three to four minutes per side.
8. Note: When turning them over, be careful because they can easily crumble.

Fruity Smoothie Bowl

Total Time Required: 10 minutes

Yields Provided: 2-4

Ingredients Needed:
- Mixed berries (1 cup)
- Burro banana (1)
- Seeded grapes (.25 cup)
- Blueberries (.25 cup)
- Strawberries (.25 cup)
- Mango (1)
- Walnut/Soft-jelly coconut milk (2-3 tbsp.)
- Nut butter - your choice - homemade tahini/walnut/Brazil nut butter (1 tbsp.)
- Date sugar or agave syrup (as desired)

Instructions:

1. Toss the berries and the banana into a blender. Pulse using the low-setting until only small bits remain.
2. Measure and mix in nut butter, a bit of soft-jelly coconut/walnut milk, and sugar or agave syrup to your liking. Use the low-setting to mix again. Be sure to scrape the sides as needed to ensure the mixture is thoroughly blended.

3. The mixture will reach a soft-serve consistency.
4. Scoop it into a bowl and top with the rest of the fruit: grapes, blueberries, strawberries, and mango as desired.

Kamut Breakfast Porridge

Total Time Required: 20 minutes
Yields Provided: 2-4

Ingredients Needed:
- Kamut (7 oz./approx. 1 cup)
- Walnut/soft-jelly coconut milk (3.75 cups)
- Sea salt (.5 tsp.)
- Coconut oil (1 tbsp.)
- Agave syrup (4 tbsp.)

Instructions:

1. On a high-speed blender or food processor, mill the Kamut until you have about 1.25 cups of cracked Kamut.
2. Combine cracked Kamut, walnut, or coconut milk, and sea salt in a pan, stirring to combine.
3. Wait for it to boil using the high-temperature setting. Adjust the temperature at med-low. Stir occasionally - until thickened as desired (10 min.).
4. Transfer the pan to a cool burner. Mix in the oil and syrup.
5. Top it off using fresh fruit as desired, and enjoy your porridge!

Kamut Alkaline Cereal – Dr.Sebi's Inspired

Total Time Required: 10 minutes
Yields Provided: 2

Ingredients Needed:
- Kamut (1 cup)
- Spring water (2 cups)
- Sea salt (1 pinch)
  Optional Seasonings:
- Cayenne
- Onion powder
- Oregano

Instructions:

1. Prepare a saucepan and bring the spring water and a tiny bit of salt to a boil.
2. Pour the berries into a food processor and grind it until it looks like grits.
3. Pour the Kamut into the boiling water and continuously stir.
4. Add spring water as needed to reach the desired consistency.
5. Sprinkle the seasonings to your liking and serve.

Strawberry Jam – Dr.Sebi's Inspired

Total Time Required: 25 minutes
Yields Provided: 16 oz.

Ingredients Needed:
- Sliced strawberries (4 cups/approx. 2 lb.)
- Raw agave (.66 or 2/3 cups)
- Key lime juice (3 tbsp.)
- Moss gel (.5 cup)

Instructions:

1. Slice enough strawberries for four cups. Mash/blend them into a chunky consistency as desired.
2. Add the strawberries, lime juice, and agave into a saucepan using the med-high temperature setting.
3. Cook for ten minutes before adding the moss gel.
4. Cook for five more minutes, stirring to ensure the gel dissolves evenly.
5. Remove from heat and wait for it to cool before refrigerating.

Veggie Omelet

Total Time Required: 15 minutes
Yields Provided: 1

Ingredients Needed:
- Spring water (.33 cup)
- Garbanzo bean flour (.25 cup)
- Cayenne powder (.25 tsp.)
- Sweet basil (.25 tsp.)
- Sea salt (.25 tsp.)
- Oregano (.25 tsp.)
- Onion powder (.25 tsp.)
- Roma tomato (.25 cup)
- Onion (.25 cup)
- Green pepper (.25 cup)
- Mushrooms (.25 cup)
- Grapeseed oil (as needed)

Instructions:

1. Dice the tomatoes, onions, peppers, and mushrooms.
2. Whisk the flour with the water and seasonings in a mixing container.
3. Pour oil (1 tsp.) into a skillet to warm using the medium-temperature setting.
4. Add a spoonful of each veggie and tomatoes to the skillet and sauté (2-3 min.).

5. Empty the "egg" mixture into the pan and cook it for three to four minutes before flipping it.
6. Slightly lift the omelet's sides and tilt the skillet towards the raised area so the mixture can get to the bottom to cook.
7. Flip the omelet and sprinkle using some of the *Brazil Nut Cheese* on half of the omelet.
8. Fold it over and serve.

Chapter 2
<u>Smoothies</u>

Dr. Sebi's smoothie recipes vary with size portions. Most of them can be for one to two servings using a high-speed blender such as a NutriBullet. Let's begin!

<u>Alkaline-Mineral Smoothie</u>

Total Time Required: 5 minutes

Ingredients Needed:
- Papaya, with seeds (half of 1 large)
- Dates (4-5)
- Burro bananas (2)
- Fresh spring water (1 cup)
- Bromide Plus Powder (1 tbsp.)
- Juice (half of 1 key lime)

Instructions:
1. Prepare the fixings. Juice the lime. Prep the bananas and papaya.
2. Toss everything into a high-speed blender.
3. Pulse and serve in chilled glasses.

The Anti-Bloat Smoothie

Total Time Required: 5 minutes

Ingredients Needed:
- Soft-jelly coconut water (.5 cup)
- Dr. Sebi's Stomach Relief Herbal Tea (.5 cup)
- Bromide Plus Powder (.5 tsp.)
- Cucumber - seeded (half of 1)
- Burro banana (1)
- High-speed blender needed

Instructions:

1. Prepare the tea and let it cool for a few minutes.
2. Mix all the components in the blender and enjoy.
3. Note: This anti-bloat smoothie will help you fight stomach bloat immediately. The tea will soothe your stomach, providing instant comfort, while the other anti-bloat ingredients start working. Cucumbers are loaded with water to help keep you remain hydrated. Burro bananas and coconut water are filled with potassium to fight water retention.

4. The Bromide Powder will give the anti-bloat smoothie the boost it needs to energize you and keep your stomach and digestion working properly.

Apple Pie Sea Moss Smoothie

Yields Provided: 2

Ingredients Needed:
- Fresh apple juice (2 cups)
- Sea Moss gel (1 heaping tbsp.)
- Fresh ginger (1 tbsp./optional)
- Clove powder (1 dash)
- Ice cubes (2 cups)

Instructions:

1. Prepare the juice and prep the ginger.
2. Toss everything into a blender.
3. Pulse until the smoothie is frothy and creamy to serve.

"Apple Pie" Smoothie

Total Time Required: 20 minutes

Ingredients Needed:
- Apple (half of 1 large)
- Figs (2)
- Small handful walnuts (1 small handful)
- Ginger tea (1 cup)
- Date sugar (1 tbsp.)
- Bromide Plus Powder (1 tsp.)

Instructions:

1. Prepare the tea and wait for it to cool.
2. Prepare the apple and walnuts. Toss everything into the blender.
3. Pulse and serve to enjoy!

Berry Heart-Healthy Smoothie

Total Time Required: 6 minutes

Ingredients Needed:
- Bromide plus Powder (1 tbsp.)
- Strawberries (.5 cup)
- Walnuts (.25 cup)
- Blueberries (.5 cup)
- Blackberries (.5 cup)
- Raspberries (.5 cup)

Instructions:

1. Measure all of the fixings.
2. Toss in a blend them using a high-speed blender.
3. Serve in cold glasses.

"Blissful" Smoothie

Total Time Required: 6-8 minutes

Ingredients Needed:
- Pear (1)
- Avocado (¼ of 1)
- Blueberries (1 oz./28 g)
- Cooked quinoa (.25 cup)
- Water (1 cup)

Instructions:

1. Chop the pear and pit the avocado—Cook the quinoa.
2. Measure the fixings and toss them into a high-speed blender.
3. Serve when it's as desired.

"Brain-Boosting" Smoothie

Total Time Required: 15 minutes + cool time

Ingredients Needed:
- Dr. Sebi's Nerve/Stress Relief Herbal Tea (.5 tbsp.) + Distilled water (1 cup)
- Raspberries (.5 cup)
- Blueberries (.5 cup)
- Burro banana (half of 1)
- Date sugar/agave syrup (1 tbsp.)

Instructions:

1. Prepare the "brain-boosting" smoothie by boiling one cup of water and add Dr. Sebi's Tea.
2. Steep the tea for 10 to 15 minutes. Strain it in a mesh sieve and wait for it to cool.
3. Once it's cooled, pour it into a high-speed blender with the rest of the ingredients.
4. Pulse to your liking and serve.

Chamomile Delight Smoothie - Dr. Sebi' Style

Total Time Required: 20-25 minutes
Ingredients Needed:
- Burro banana (1)
- Prepared Nerve/Stress Relief Herbal Tea (.25 cup)
- Homemade walnut milk (.5 cup)
- Date sugar (1 tbsp.)

Instructions:

1. Prepare the tea and wait for it to cool before adding it to the blender.
2. Mix in the rest of the fixings and pulse until it's creamy to your liking.

Dr. Sebi's Blueberry Smoothie

Total Time Required: 15 minutes for the quinoa + 5 minutes prep

Ingredients Needed:
- Cooked quinoa (.25 cup)
- Blueberries (.5 cup)
- Homemade walnut milk (1 cup)
- Burro banana (1)
- Date sugar (2 tbsp.)

Instructions:

1. Rinse the berries—Cook the quinoa.
2. Toss each of the fixings into a high-speed blender.
3. Serve and garnish as desired.

Dr. Sebi's Blueberry-Pie Smoothie

Total Time Required: 10 minutes

Ingredients Needed:
- Fresh blueberries (1 cup)
- Burro banana (1)
- Homemade soft-jelly coconut milk (2 cups)
- Cooked amaranth (.25 cup)
- Bromide Plus Powder (1 tsp.)
- Homemade walnut butter (1 tbsp.)
- Date sugar (2 tbsp.)

Instructions:

1. Mix each of the fixings in a blender such as NutriBullet.
2. Allow the smoothie to solidify in the freezer until ready to drink.

<u>Dr. Sebi's Classic Detox Smoothie</u>

Total Time Required: 20 minutes

Ingredients Needed:
- Burro banana (½ of 1)
- Romaine lettuce (1 cup)
- Key lime juice (2 - 3 tbsp.)
- Ginger tea (.5 cup)
- Blueberries (.25 cup)
- Soft jelly coconut water (.5 cup)

Instructions:

1. This is excellent to begin a cleanse.
2. Prep the banana and berries. Make the tea and wait for it to steep.
3. Add the fixings into a blender and mix.
4. Serve when ready.

Dr. Sebi's Detox Berry Smoothie

Total Time Required: 10 minutes

Ingredients Needed:
- Medium burro banana (1)
- Seville orange (1)
- Blueberries or a mixture of blueberries - strawberries & raspberries (1 cup)
- Fresh lettuce (2 cups)
- Hemp seeds (1 tbsp.)
- Water
- Pitted avocado (¼ of 1)

Instructions:

1. Add the water to your blender first, followed by the fruit and the greens.

Blend all of the ingredients until smooth and creamy as desired.

<u>Dr. Sebi's Energizer Smoothie</u>

Total Time Required: 10 minutes

Ingredients Needed:
- Papaya or melon (1 cup)
- Homemade hemp milk (1 cup)
- Cooked quinoa or amaranth (.5 cup)
- Date (1) or Date sugar (1 tbsp.)
- Bromide Plus Powder (1 tsp.)

Instructions:

1. Chop the melon into cubes and cook the quinoa.
2. Toss the cooled fixings into the high-powered blender.
3. Pulse and serve in a chilled glass.

Dr. Sebi's Green Detox Smoothie

Total Time Required: 20 minutes

Ingredients Needed:
- Burro banana (half of 1)
- Romaine lettuce (1 cup)
- Key lime juice (2-3 tbsp.)
- Ginger tea (.5 cup)
- Blueberries (.25 cup)
- Soft jelly coconut water (.5 cup)

Instructions:

1. Make the tea and let it cool.
2. Toss each of the fixings into the NutriBullet or another blender.
3. Pulse until creamy to serve.

Dr. Sebi's Heart-Healthy Smoothie

Total Time Required: 5 minutes

Ingredients Needed:
- Braeburn apple, or another kind of organic apple (1)
- Brazil nuts (.25 cup)
- Homemade walnut milk (1 cup)
- Blueberries (1 cup)
- Approved greens - ex. - Dandelion greens, watercress, turnip greens, etc. (1 cup)
- Date sugar or agave syrup (.5 tbsp.)

Instructions:

1. Toss the fixings into your high-speed blender.
2. Pulse until incorporated and serve.

Dr. Sebi's Herbal Smoothie

Total Time Required: 15 minutes

Ingredients Needed:
- Dr. Sebi's Herbal Tea (your favorite)
- Walnuts
- Burro banana (1)
- Date sugar or agave syrup (1 tbsp.)

Instructions:

1. Prepare the tea according to the package directions. Let it cool.
2. Blend the tea with the burro banana, walnuts, and date sugar or agave syrup in a high-speed blender.
3. Serve in a chilled glass/glasses.

Dr. Sebi's Hormone-Balancing Smoothie

Total Time Required: 5-6 minutes

Ingredients Needed:
- Homemade walnut milk (1.25 cups)
- Zucchini (.33 cup)
- Avocado (¼ of 1)
- Dandelion greens (2 handfuls)
- Hemp seeds (3 tbsp.)

Instructions:

1. Dice the zucchini. Refer to the recipe for walnut milk in chapter one.
2. So easy to toss them into the high-speed blender.
3. Serve when it's as desired.

Dr. Sebi's Creamy Relaxing Smoothie

Total Time Required: 20 minutes

Ingredients Needed:
- Prepared Dr. Sebi's Nerve/Stress Relief Herbal Tea** (.5 cup)
- Burro banana (1)
- Avocado (¼ of 1)
- Seeded cucumber (¼ of 1)
- Soft-jelly coconut milk (1 cup)
- Chopped walnuts (1 tbsp.)
- Optional: Date sugar/agave syrup (1 tbsp.)

Instructions:

1. Boil two cups of distilled water and add one (1) tablespoon of Herbal Tea**.
2. Steep for 10 to 15 minutes, strain, and let the tea cool.
3. Blend half a cup of the tea with the remainder of the fixings in a high-speed blender.
4. Adjust sweetness as needed and serve.

Dr. Sebi's Iron Power Smoothie

Total Time Required: 8-10 minutes

Ingredients Needed:
- Large red apple (half of 1)
- Currants or raisins (1 tbsp.)
- Fig (1)
- Cooked quinoa (.5 cup)
- Homemade hemp seed milk (1 cup)
- Amaranth greens (2 handfuls)
- Date sugar (1 tbsp.)
- Bromide Plus Powder (1 tsp.)

Instructions:

1. Prepare the quinoa beforehand.
2. Measure the fixings and toss them into a high-powered blender.
3. Pulse until creamy smooth to serve.

Dr. Sebi's Relaxation Smoothie

Total Time Required: 10-15 minutes

Ingredients Needed:
- Cantaloupe (1 cup)
- Zucchini (1)
- Burro banana (half of 1)
- Nerve/Stress Relief Herbal Tea (.5 cup)
- Soft-jelly coconut water (.5 cup)

Instructions:

1. Prepare the tea according to instructions and let it cool.
2. Chop the zucchini. Prep the banana into chunks.
3. Combine each of the fixings, including the tea, in a blender.
4. Pour in a cup or two and enjoy.

Dr. Sebi's "Veggie-Ful" Smoothie

Total Time Required: 5 minutes

Ingredients Needed:
- Pear (1)
- Avocado (¼ of 1)
- Cucumber (half of 1)
- Watercress (1 handful)
- Romaine lettuce (1 handful)
- Spring water (.5 cup)
- Optional: Date sugar (as desired)

Instructions:

1. Core and remove the seeds from the pear and seeds from the cucumber.
2. Blend each of the fixings in a blender, pulsing until it's creamy.
3. Serve in chilled mugs.

Energy-Boosting - Dr. Sebi's Green Smoothie

Total Time Required: 8-10 minutes

Ingredients Needed:
- Greens - dandelion greens, amaranth greens, lettuce, or wild arugula (2 handfuls)
- Seeded cucumber (half of 1)
- Apple (1)
- Burro banana (1)
- Bromide Plus Powder (.5 tsp.)
- Walnuts (1 tbsp.)
- Soft-jelly coconut milk (1 cup)

Instructions:

1. Make the smoothie by blending all of the fixings in a high-speed processor.
2. Serve in a tall chilled glass.

The Glowing Green Smoothie

Total Time Required: 5-8 minutes

Ingredients Needed:
- Approved greens (2 cups)
- Pear (half of 1)
- Braeburn or another kind of organic apple (half of 1)
- Burro banana (half of 1)
- Seeded cucumber (half of 1)
- Key lime (1 juiced)
- Cayenne pepper (1 pinch)
- Optional: Spring water/soft-jelly coconut water (2 cups)

Instructions:

1. Chop and measure all of the fixings before starting to make it much easier.
2. Toss them into your high-speed blender.
3. Pulse and serve in chilled glasses.

Heavy Metal Detox Smoothie

Total Time Required: 5-6 minutes

Ingredients Needed:
- Burro banana (1)
- Blueberries (1-2 cups)
- Seville orange juice (1 cup)
- Watercress (1 cup)
- Organic apple (1)
- Dr. Sebi's Bromide Plus Powder (1 tbsp.)
- Springwater (1 cup)

Instructions:

1. Prepare the heavy metal smoothie by tossing all of its components in a blender until it's creamy.
2. You can add up to one cup of water to reach a less thick smoothie if desired.

Immunity-Boosting Smoothie

Total Time Required: 25 minutes

Ingredients Needed:
- Mango (half of 1)
- Seville orange (1)
- Brewed Dr. Sebi's Immune Support Herbal Tea (1 cup)
- Coconut oil (1 tbsp.)
- Date sugar or agave syrup (1 tbsp.)
- Key lime (1 juiced)

Instructions:

1. Boil distilled water (2 cups) and add 1.5 tablespoons of Dr. Sebi's Herbal Tea. Simmer for about 15 minutes. Allow to cool, strain.
2. Peel the Seville orange and cut the mango into chunks.
3. Mix all the fixings in a blender.

Magnesium-Boosting Smoothie

Total Time Required: 20 minutes

Ingredients Needed:
- Fresh spring water (1 cup)
- Brazil Nuts (.25 cup)
- Burro banana (half of 1)
- Strawberries (2)
- Figs (.5 cup)
- Optional: Dr. Sebi's Bromide Plus Powder (1 tsp.)

Instructions:

1. Blend each of the fixings in a blender.
2. Mix in a tiny bit of water as desired for thinning the smoothie.
3. Boost the magnesium content of the smoothie by adding the Bromide. The powder acts as a natural diuretic. It suppresses the appetite, regulates bowels, and it's helpful in the overall digestive system.

Mood-Boosting Smoothie

Total Time Required: 20-25 minutes

Ingredients Needed:
- Nerve/Stress Relief Herbal Tea (1 cup)
- Soft-jelly coconut meat (.5 cup)
- Strawberries (1 cup)
- Date sugar/agave syrup (as desired)
- Suggested: High-speed blender

Instructions:

1. To prepare the mood-booster, begin by boiling one cup of distilled water and add ½ tablespoon of Dr. Sebi's Tea. Steep for 10 to 15 minutes, strain. Let it cool.
2. Blend the tea with the remainder of the fixings in the blender.
3. Serve as desired.

Orange Creamsicle Smoothie

Total Time Required: 5-6 minutes

Ingredients Needed:
- Seville oranges (3)
- Burro banana (half of 1)
- Coconut water (1 cup)
- Date sugar (as desired)
- Bromide Plus Powder (.5 tsp.)

Instructions:

1. Peel the oranges and prep the banana.
2. Add each of the fixings into the blender.
3. Pulse until smooth and serve.

Original "Bromide-Plus" Smoothie

Total Time Required: 5-6 minutes

Ingredients Needed:
- Bromide Plus Powder (.5 tbsp.)
- Agave syrup (.25 cup)
- Fresh (approved) fruit (1 cup)
- Boiling spring water (1 quart)
- Walnuts (3 tbsp.)

Instructions:

1. Combine the agave syrup, fruit, walnuts, and Bromide Powder in the blender.
2. Slowly, pour in the quart of water, and blend for three to four minutes.
3. Let it cool, and serve.

Pancreas-Support Smoothie Specialty

Total Time Required: 20 minutes

Ingredients Needed:
- Dr. Sebi's Stomach Relief Herbal Tea (2 cups)
- Tamarind pulp (1 tbsp.)
- Seeded cucumber (1)
- Watercress or wild arugula (1 fistful)
- Juice - key lime (1)

Instructions:

1. To prepare your smoothie, begin by boiling two cups of distilled water with 1½ tablespoons of herbal tea.
2. Simmer for about 15 minutes—strain and cool.
3. Blend the tea with the rest of the components in a high-speed blender.
4. Serve when it's to your liking.

Seibi Inspired Peach Berry Smoothie

Total Time Required: 5 minutes
Yields Provided: 2

Ingredients Needed:
Use frozen fruit (.5 cup each):
- Peaches
- Cherries
- Blueberries
- Strawberries
- Coconut water (1 cup)
- Hemp seeds (1 tbsp.)
- Agave (1 tbsp.)
- Sea Moss Gel (1 tbsp.)

Instructions:

1. Add all ingredients to a blender. Combine for one minute.
2. If it needs to be thinner, mix in coconut water (up to another ¼ of a cup), and blend for another 20 seconds.

"Stomach Soother" Smoothie

Total Time Required: 20 minutes

Ingredients Needed:
- Burro banana (1)
- Prepared Dr. Sebi's Stomach Relief Herbal Tea (.5 cup)
- Ginger tea (.5 cup)
- Agave syrup (1 tbsp.)

Instructions:

1. Prepare tea as instructed and let cool.
2. Blend with the remaining ingredients and serve in a chilled mug.

Sugar-Detox Smoothie

Total Time Required: 6-7 minutes

Ingredients Needed:
- Avocado (half of 1)
- Homemade soft-jelly coconut milk (1 cup)
- "Approved" greens - ex. callaloo, watercress, or dandelion greens (1 handful)
- Key lime (1 squeeze)
- Dr. Sebi's Bromide Plus Powder (1 tsp.)

Instructions:

1. Prepare a high-speed blender. Toss in the fixings.
2. Serve when it's as desired.

Super Hydrating Smoothie

Total Time Required: 5 minutes

Ingredients Needed:
- Strawberries (1 cup)
- Watermelon chunks (1 cup)
- Soft jelly coconut water (1 cup)
- Date sugar (1 tbsp.)

Instructions:

1. Toss each of the fixings together in the blender.
2. Serve in a chilled glass.

Sweet Sunrise Smoothie

Total Time Required: 6-8 minutes

Ingredients Needed:
- Raspberries (1 cup)
- Seville orange (1)
- Burro banana (half of 1)
- Mango (1 cup)
- Water (1 cup)

Instructions:

1. Toss the ingredients into the blender.
2. Set it to high-speed or use a NutriBullet.
3. Pulse and serve in a chilled glass.

Triple Berry Smoothie

Total Time Required: 5 minutes

Ingredients Needed:
- Blueberries (.5 cup)
- Strawberries (.5 cup)
- Burro banana (1)
- Raspberries (.5 cup)
- Agave syrup (as desired)
- Water (1 cup)

Directions:

1. Toss the fixings into a high-speed blender such as NutriBullet.
2. Serve in a chilled glass.

"Tropical Breeze" Smoothie

Total Time Required: 8-10 minutes

Ingredients Needed:
- Mango (half of 1)
- Cantaloupe (.5 cup)
- Watermelon (.5 cup)
- Burro banana (half of 1)
- Soft jelly coconut water (1 cup)
- Amaranth greens (1 handful)

Instructions:

1. Prepare the cantaloupe, mango, watermelon, and banana.
2. Toss it all into the high-powered blender and pulse.
3. Serve in a cold glass.

Chapter 3
Lunch & Dinner Salad Favorites

Alkaline-Electric Spring Salad

Total Time Required: 8-10 minutes
Yields Provided: 4-6

Ingredients Needed:
- Seasonal approved greens of your choice - wild arugula, dandelion greens, watercress (4 cups)
- Cherry tomatoes (1 cup)
- Walnuts (.25 cup)
- Approved herbs of your choice - dill, sweet basil, etc. (.25 cup)
  The Dressing:
- Key limes (3-4)
- Homemade raw sesame "tahini" butter (1 tbsp.)
- Sea salt & cayenne pepper (as desired)

Instructions:

1. Juice the key limes.

2. Whisk the key lime juice with the homemade raw sesame "tahini" butter. Add sea salt and cayenne.
3. Slice the cherry tomatoes into halves.
4. Toss the greens, tomatoes, and herbs into a big mixing container.
5. Empty the dressing over the top and "massage" the salad with your hands.
6. Let the greens soak up the dressing.
7. Add seasonings and herbs as desired.

Asian Cucumber Salad

Total Time Required: 5-6 minutes
Yields Provided: 1

Ingredients Needed:
- Sesame oil (1 tbsp.)
- Key lime juice (3 tbsp.)
- Date sugar (.5 tsp.)
- Grated ginger (1 tbsp.)
- Sea salt (.25 tsp.)
- Sesame seeds (1 tbsp.)
- Powdered granulated seaweed (1 tbsp.)

Instructions:

1. Toss each of the fixings into a salad container to serve.

Basil Avocado Pasta Salad

Total Time Required: 15 minutes
Yields Provided: 1-2

Ingredients Needed:
- Avocado (1)
- Fresh basil (1 cup)
- Cherry tomatoes (1 pint)
- Key lime juice (1 tbsp.)
- Olive oil (.25 cup)
- Agave syrup (1 tsp.)
- Spelt-pasta - cooked (4 cups)

Instructions:

1. Toss the cooked pasta in a big mixing container.
2. Slice the tomatoes into halves.
3. Chop and add avocado with chopped basil and tomatoes.
4. Thoroughly stir until incorporated.
5. Whisk the oil with lime juice, agave syrup, and sea salt.
6. Pour over pasta and stir to combine.
7. **** You can use another type of pasta, but it must be approved by Dr. Sebi's Cell Food.

Cherry Tomato Salad

Total Time Required: 10 minutes
Yields Provided: 2-4

Ingredients Needed:
- Cherry tomatoes (4 cups)
- Red onion (.25 cup)
- Fresh (approved) herbs such as dill, sweet basil, or thyme (.25 cup)
- Olive oil (.25 cup)
- Key lime juice (1.5 tbsp.)
- Date sugar (.25 tsp.)
- Salt & Cayenne pepper (as desired)

Instructions:

1. To prepare your cherry tomato salad, chop the onion and prep the desired herbs.
2. Start by placing the tomatoes, red onion, and herbs in a big mixing container.
3. Prepare the dressing by whisking the oil with the juice, sea salt, date sugar, and cayenne pepper as desired.
4. Sprinkle the dressing over the tomato mixture, gently tossing to coat evenly. Serve.

Dandelion Strawberry Salad

Total Time Required: 20 minutes
Yields Provided: 1-2

Ingredients Needed:
- Grapeseed oil (2 tbsp.)
- Medium red onion (1)
- Ripe strawberries (10)
- Key lime juice (2 tbsp.)
- Dandelion greens (4 cups)
- Sea salt (as desired)
- Suggested: 12-inch skillet

Instructions:

1. Prep the skillet with oil using the medium-temperature setting.
2. Slice and add the onions with a generous pinch of sea salt.
3. Sauté them often stirring until they're softened, lightly brown, and reduced to about 1/3 of its raw volume.
4. Slice and toss the strawberry with one teaspoon of juice.
5. Rinse the dandelion greens and chop them into bite-sized pieces.
6. When the onions are nearly done, add the rest of the lime juice to the pan. Continue

cooking until it has thickened to coat the onions (1-2 min.).

7. Remove the onions from the hot burner.
8. Toss the greens, onions, and strawberries with all their juices.
9. Sprinkle with sea salt to serve.

<u>Detox Salad Burritos</u>

Total Time Required: 35-40 minutes
Yields Provided: 4

Ingredients Needed:
- Wild arugula, or other approved greens (2 cups)
- Cherry tomatoes (2 cups)
- Homemade raw sesame "tahini" butter (2 tbsp.)
- Key lime juice (1 tbsp.)
- Cooked chickpeas or garbanzo beans (1 cup)
- Kamut flour tortillas (4)
- Sea salt & cayenne pepper (as desired)

Instructions:

1. In a small cup, prepare the dressing by whisking key lime juice and raw sesame "tahini" butter. Set it to the side.
2. Toss the wild arugula, cherry tomatoes, and chickpeas. Cover with the dressing and let the flavors meld for 20 minutes in the fridge.
3. Use a big skillet or griddle using a low-temperature setting to warm the tortillas until they are pliable.
4. Fill the tortillas with the salad, cayenne, and sea salt; roll 'em up.

Detox Watercress Citrus Delight Salad

Total Time Required: 5-10 minutes
Yields Provided: 1-2

Ingredients Needed:
- Avocado - ripe (1)
- Watercress (4 cups)
- Seville orange (1)
- Red onion (2)
- Key lime juice (2 tbsp.)
- Agave syrup (2 tsp.)
- Olive oil (2 tbsp.)
- Salt (.125 or ⅛ tsp.)
- Optional: Cayenne pepper

Instructions:

1. Peel, slice, and zest the orange. Thinly slice the onion.
2. Arrange watercress, avocado, onion, and oranges on two plates.
3. Whisk the lime juice with the salt, oil, agave, and cayenne in a small mixing container.
4. Spoon dressing over salad when ready to serve.

Dr. Sebi's Fall Pear Walnut Salad

Total Time Required: 15 minutes
Yields Provided: 2

Ingredients Needed:
- Walnut halves (.5 cup)
- Agave syrup (.25 cup)
- Sea salt (1 pinch)
- Wild arugula (8 large handfuls)
- Pears (2 large)
- Olive oil (4 tbsp.)
- Key lime juice (.25 cup)

Instructions:

1. Warm the oven to reach 350° Fahrenheit or 177° Celsius.
2. Mix the walnuts with one tablespoon of agave syrup and a pinch of sea salt. Spread out on a lined baking tray and bake until golden (7-8 min.).
3. Transfer the pan to the countertop to cool.
4. Add the rest of the agave syrup, lime juice, oil, and a pinch of the sea salt to a small jar. Place the top securely on the jar and thoroughly shake it.
5. Gently wash the pears and halve them lengthways. Remove the cores with a

teaspoon. Then cut each half into long thin slices.

6. Add the arugula and sliced pear to a large salad bowl.
7. Sprinkle over the cooled walnuts and drizzle generously with the dressing just before serving.

Dr. Sebi's Headache Preventing Salad

Total Time Required: 5-10 minutes
Yields Provided: 1-2

Ingredients Needed:
- Cucumber (half of 1 - seeded)
- Watercress (2 cups)
- Olive oil (2 tbsp.)
- Key lime juice (1 tbsp.)
- Salt & cayenne (to your liking)

Instructions:

1. Rinse the veggies.
2. Whisk the oil and juice until thoroughly combined.
3. Arrange watercress and cucumber.
4. Add the dressing and dusting of pepper and salt to serve.

Dr. Sebi's Roasted Quinoa Salad

Total Time Required: 40 minutes
Yields Provided: 4

Ingredients Needed:
- Vegetable homemade broth (2.5 cups)
- Sea salt (2 tsp.)
- Quinoa (2 cups)
- Green bell peppers (2)
- Red bell pepper (1)
- Zucchini (1)
- Grapeseed oil (2 tbsp.)
- Sea salt
- Wild arugula/another approved green (3 cups)
- Avocado (1)
- Red onion (1/to taste)

Instructions:

1. Set the oven to 400° Fahrenheit/204° Celsius.
2. Slice the green peppers into halves - lengthwise.
3. Core and dice the red pepper. Chop the zucchini into small chunks as desired.
4. Simmer the broth and salt using the medium-temperature setting. Stir in the quinoa.

5. Once simmering, lower the temperature setting to low. Place a top on the pot.
6. Simmer for 20 minutes and extinguish the heat. Let it sit until serving time.
7. Before serving, fluff the quinoa using a fork.
8. While the quinoa is simmering, add bell peppers and zucchini to a big sheet pan. Gently toss them using oil and a dusting of salt as desired.
9. Roast until everything is golden and tender (10-12 min.).
10. Toss the fixings and garnish with onion and avocado as you fold in the quinoa to serve.

The Grilled Romaine Lettuce Salad

Total Time Required: 20 minutes
Yields Provided: 1-2

Ingredients Needed:
- Romaine lettuce (4 small heads)
- Red onion (1 tbsp.)
- Key lime juice (1 tbsp.)
- Fresh basil (1 tbsp.)
- Onion powder + cayenne pepper + sea salt (to your liking)
- Olive oil (4 tbsp.)
- Agave syrup (1 tbsp.)

Instructions:

1. Thoroughly rinse the lettuce. Finely chop the onion and basil. Juice the lime.
2. Arrange the lettuce halves cut side down in a large nonstick pan. Don't add any oil. Check the color of the lettuce by turning them. Make sure the lettuce is browned equally on each side.
3. Scoop it onto a large platter or baking tray to cool.
4. For the dressing, combine the onion with olive oil, agave syrup, lime juice, salt,

cayenne, and fresh basil in a mixing container. Whisk it thoroughly to combine.

5. Transfer the grilled lettuce onto a serving dish and drizzle with the dressing to serve.

Roasted Vegetable Winter Salad

Total Time Required: 30 minutes
Yields Provided: 4-6

Ingredients Needed:
- Zucchinis (4 small)
- Red bell peppers (2)
- Cherry tomatoes (1 cup)
- Red onion (1 large)
- Mushrooms (1 cup)
- Grapeseed oil (.25 cup)
- Dr. Sebi's approved herbs (2 tbsp.)
- Sea salt and cayenne pepper (as desired)
- Suggested: Rimmed baking sheet

Instructions:

1. Warm the oven to 425° Fahrenheit/218° Celsius.
2. Cut the zucchini and the large red onion into thick wedges. Cut the cherry tomatoes and mushrooms in half, and slice the red bell pepper.
3. Place the vegetables on the baking tray with a spritz of grapeseed oil, sea salt, cayenne pepper, and herbs - toss to combine. Spread out in an even layer.

4. Roast until tender and lightly caramelized, stirring halfway through, about 20 minutes total.

Mango Salad - Dr. Sebi Style

Total Time Required: 30 minutes
Yields Provided: 2-4

Ingredients Needed:
- Mangoes (2)
- Red onion (¼ of 1)
- Cherry tomatoes (.25 cup)
- Cucumber (half of 1 - seeded)
- Green bell pepper (half of 1)
- Key lime (1)
- Sea salt & cayenne pepper (to your liking)

Instructions:

1. To prepare your salad, start by cutting the mangoes, cherry tomatoes, and red onion into small cubes.
2. Slice the seeded cucumber and the bell pepper finely.
3. Combine all of the fixings in a mixing container with salt and pepper as desired. Juice the key lime and pour over the salad.
4. Marinate in the fridge for at least 20 minutes before eating.
5. Enjoy as a salad, salsa, or dip.

Wakame Salad

Total Time Required: 20 minutes
Yields Provided: 1

Ingredients Needed:
- Wakame stems/other sea vegetables from Dr. Sebi's Guide (2 cups)
- Agave syrup (1 tbsp.)
- Sesame oil (1 tbsp.)
- Ginger (1 tsp.)
- Bell pepper - red (1 tbsp.)
- Sesame seeds (1 tbsp.)
- Onion powder (1 tsp.)
- Key lime juice (1 tbsp.)

Instructions:

1. Soak the wakame stems for five to ten minutes and drain.
2. Whisk the sesame oil with the agave syrup, onion powder, key lime juice, and ginger.
3. Place the wakame and bell pepper in a serving dish. Pour dressing on top.
4. Sprinkle with sesame seeds and serve.

Chapter 4
Lunch & Dinner Meals

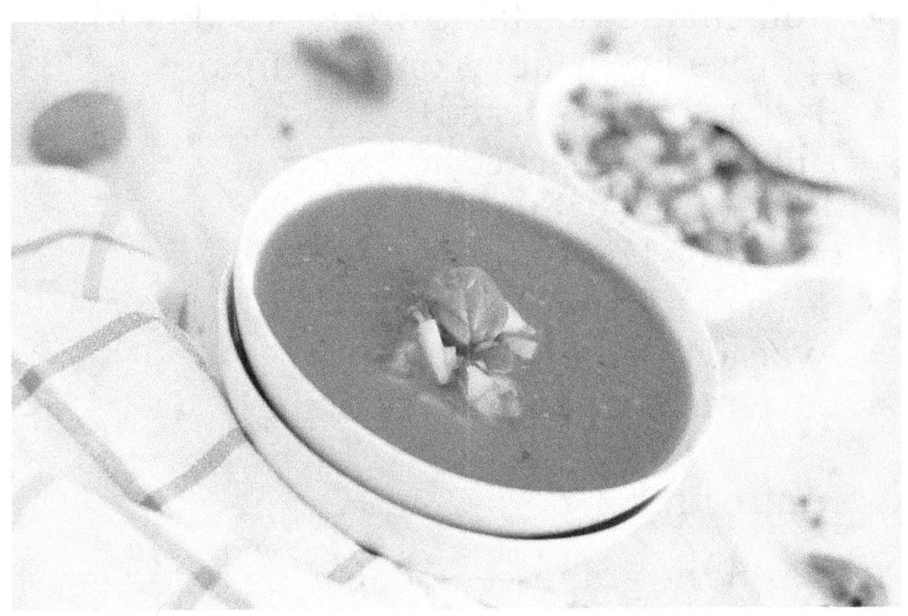

Soup Options

Cleansing Green Soup

Total Time Required: 60 minutes
Yields Provided: 4

Ingredients Needed:

- Yellow onions, peeled and roughly chopped (3 medium or 2 large)
- Zucchini (1)
- Dandelion greens (1 bunch)
- Wild arugula (1 bunch)
- Homemade vegetable broth - made with approved vegetables only (4 cups)
- Basil (.5 cup - packed)
- Dill (.5 cup - packed)
- Juice of 1 key lime
- Grapeseed oil (3 tbsp.)
- Sea salt (.25 tsp.)
- Avocado (¼ of 1)
- Cayenne pepper (to your liking)

Instructions:

1. Warm the grapeseed oil in a big pot using the med-high temperature setting until warm.
2. Rinse, peel and roughly chop the onions. Rinse and chop the zucchini.
3. Toss in the onions and simmer for five minutes, occasionally stirring, until translucent.
4. Add dandelion greens, zucchini, and wild arugula, and cook (5 min.).

5. Mix in the vegetable stock. Wait for it to boil and adjust the setting to low. Place a top on the pot and simmer (15-20 min.).
6. Let cool, uncovered (15 min.).
7. If necessary, working in batches - blend with basil, avocado, dill, key lime juice, sea salt, and cayenne pepper until very smooth.
8. Serve and adjust seasonings. Decorate with fresh herbs.

Cream of Mushroom Soup

Total Time Required: 35-40 minutes
Yields Provided: 6

Ingredients Needed:
- Grapeseed oil (2 tbsp.)
- Onion (1)
- Mushrooms - cremini or white (2 lb./910 g)
- Fresh thyme (1 tbsp.) or Dried (1.5 tsp.)
- Homemade approved vegetable broth (4 cups)
- Spelt flour (3 tbsp.)
- Homemade walnut milk (1.5 cups)
- Your favorite approved herbs (.25 cup)
- Sea salt & cayenne pepper (as desired)

Instructions:

1. Warm the oil using the medium-temperature setting.
2. Dice the onion and sauté them for five minutes. Slice and toss in the mushrooms and thyme and simmer (5 min.).
3. Pour in the broth. Wait for it to boil. Put a lid on the pot and lower the temperature setting to simmer (15 min.).

4. For the last five minutes, mix in the milk and continue cooking.
5. Mix the spelt flour with cool water. Add to the soup and frequently stir until the soup slightly thickens (1-2 min.).
6. Serve with a dusting of salt and cayenne pepper to your liking.

Creamy Vegetable Soup

Total Time Required: 25-30 minutes
Yields Provided: 1

Ingredients Needed:
- Grapeseed oil (1 tbsp.)
- Bell pepper (1 red)
- Zucchini (1)
- Yellow onion (¼ of 1)
- Sea salt & Cayenne pepper (as desired)
- Optional: Approved herbs
- Homemade walnut milk (see recipe - 1 cup)

Instructions:

1. Chop and sauté the onion in the grapeseed oil until the onion is translucent.
2. Mix in the chopped pepper and zucchini. Simmer using the medium-temperature setting (5 min.).
3. When the vegetables are soft, blend with the milk.
4. Simmer for 15 minutes—season to taste.
5. Serve with fresh Dr. Sebi approved herbs.

Cucumber-Basil Gazpacho

Total Time Required: 2 hours - varies
Yields Provided: 2-4

Ingredients Needed:
- Ripe avocado (1)
- Cucumber (1)
- Fresh basil (2 small handfuls)
- Water (2 cups)
- Sea salt (1.25 tsp.)
- Juiced key lime (1)

Instructions:

1. It is okay to leave the peeling on the cucumber but discard the seeds. Juice the lime.
2. To prepare, refrigerate all ingredients until cold.
3. Toss them into a blender and purée until smooth, allowing a few specks of green to remain throughout.
4. Return the soup to the fridge and chill until ready to serve.
5. Garnish with thinly sliced cucumber circles and basil leaves.

Cucumber-Melon Soup

Total Time Required: 1 hour to overnight
Yields Provided: Varies
- Cucumbers (450 g/1 lb. + more for serving)
- Honeydew melon (half of 1 small/1 lb./450 g)
- Fresh key lime juice (1 tbsp.)
- Date sugar (2 tsp.)
- Sea salt & cayenne pepper
- To Serve: Watercress
- Suggested: High-speed blender

Instructions:

1. Slice and remove the seeds from the cucumbers and melon (rind removed).
2. Blend the cucumbers, melon, herbs, key lime juice, date sugar, and sea salt (.5 tsp.) until smooth.
3. Refrigerate for at a minimum of one hour, but it's suggested to rest overnight. Serve topped with sliced cucumber, watercress, and cayenne pepper.
4. Enjoy the soup with slices of 'approved' grain bread topped with avocado slices.

<u>Dr. Sebi's Inspired Vegetable Broth -Stew – Soup</u>

Total Time Required: 2¼ hours
Yields Provided: 4-6 cups

Ingredients Needed:
- Aquafaba - chickpea water (4 cups)
- Spring water (4 cups)
- Bell peppers - red and green (1 cup)
- Onions - red and white (1 cup)
- Mushrooms (1.5 cups)
- Butternut squash (2 cups)
- Kale (1 cup)
- Plum tomatoes (2)
- Green onions (.5 cup)
- Dill (1 tsp.)
- Cayenne powder (.5 tsp.)
- Onion powder (1 tsp.)
- Basil (1 tsp.)
- Sage (1 tsp.)
- Sea salt (1 tsp.)
- Savory (1 tsp.)
- Oregano (1 tsp.)
- Grapeseed oil

Instructions:

1. Slice/chop the onions, peppers, and mushrooms. Chop the squash, tomatoes, and kale (stems too).
2. Pour oil (about 1 tbsp.) into a stockpot to sauté the mushrooms, onions, and peppers (5 min.).
3. Mix in aquafaba, seasonings, water, and all of the other fixings into the pot. Wait for it to boil.
4. Adjust the temperature setting to low and simmer (1-2 hrs.)
5. Let the broth cool. Strain the veggies, and it's ready. You can also save the broth in glass jars to use another time.
6. Note: *If you do not have aquafaba, you can substitute using four additional cups of spring water.

Immunity-Boosting Soup

Total Time Required: 30 minutes
Yields Provided: 2-4

Ingredients Needed:
- Onion (half of 1)
- Bell pepper (1)
- Mushrooms - any kind, except shiitake (1 cup)
- Grapeseed oil (1 tbsp.)
- Approved-flour noodles - spelt, amaranth, wild rice, etc. (1 pack)
- Key lime (1)
- Zucchini (1)
- Cherry tomatoes (1 cup)
- Water (4 cups)
- Approved herbs
- Sea salt and cayenne pepper

Instructions:

1. Prepare the noodles following the package directions (8-10 min.).
2. Chop the onion into small cubes. In a big skillet, warm the grapeseed oil. Sauté the onion until it's translucent.

3. Chop the mushroom, bell pepper, and cherry tomatoes into small pieces. Sauté in the pan as well.
4. Grate the zucchini and add it to the pan.
5. Add the water, sea salt, pepper, and spices. Wait for it to boil using the medium-temperature setting.
6. Once the boiling point is reached, lower the heat. Add the cooked noodles. Let simmer for another ten minutes.
7. Adjust seasoning. Serve topped with more herbs and key lime juice.

Mighty Powerful Healing Soup - Super for Detox or Fasting

Total Time Required: 1-2 hours
Yields Provided: 1-2

Ingredients Needed:
- Approved sea vegetables (1 handful)
- Approved greens (wild arugula, lettuce, purslane, verdolaga (1 handful)
- Dandelion greens (1 cup)
- Mushrooms (any kind, except shiitake (1 cup)
- Your preferred approved herbs (.25 cup)

Instructions:

1. To prepare your "powerful healing" soup, start by simmering the detoxifying ingredients for one to two hours over a low flame.
2. Strain to drink as a broth, or if you prefer, leave the cut vegetables intact and enjoy a bowl.

Native Soup

Total Time Required: 1 hour 20 minutes
Yields Provided: 6-8

Ingredients Needed:
- Sea salt (2 tbsp.)
- Basil (2 tbsp.)
- Green & red bell pepper (1 cup of each)
- Cayenne pepper (2 tsp.)
- Oregano (2 tsp.)
- Spring water (1 gallon)
- Yellow squash
- Red onion
- Dill (1 tsp.)
- Grapeseed oil (2 tbsp.)
- Butternut squash (2 cups)
- Roma tomatoes (3)
- Zucchini
- Mushrooms (4 cups)
- Quinoa (1 cup)
- Cooked garbanzo beans (1 lb.)
- Kamut pasta (2-4 cups)

Instructions:

1. Soak the garbanzos overnight. Cook them before adding them to the soup.
2. Dice the tomatoes. Chop the onions, zucchini,

mushrooms, butternut and yellow squash, and peppers.

3. Add the water to a large pot and let it heat using the medium-temperature setting. As the water warms up, gather the prepared veggies and add them into the water.

4. Add the seasoning and wait for the soup to simmer for about one hour. Stir it frequently, and lastly, add in the beans. Stir until heated and serve.

Roasted Vegetable & Coconut Milk Soup

Total Time Required: 1 hour 20 minutes
Yields Provided: 2-4

Ingredients Needed:
- Cayenne pepper & sea salt (as desired
- Grapeseed oil (1 tbsp. + more for the veggies)
- Grated ginger (1 tbsp.)
- Coconut milk (1 cup)
- Veggies of choice (2 chopped cups)

Instructions:

1. Set the oven temperature setting to reach 350° Fahrenheit/177° Celsius.
2. Toss the chopped veggies onto a baking tray and toss thoroughly to coat—dust with pepper and salt.
3. Toss them in the oven for 40 minutes.
4. Meanwhile, prepare the sauce. Add the grapeseed oil to a skillet. Toss in the onion and saute until it's translucent. Mince and add the ginger and sauté.
5. Pour in the coconut milk and wait for it to boil.
6. Lower the temperature setting and continue to simmer for about ½ hour.

7. Once the veggies are done cooking, remove them from the oven. Pour the milk mixture into two boils and divide the veggies evenly in between the two bowls to serve.

Soursop Ginger Soup

Total Time Required: 1.5 hours
Yields Provided: 6-8

Ingredients Needed:
- Soursop Leaves (4-6)
- Spring water (12-16 cups/approx. 1 gallon)
- Kale (2 cups)
- Chayote squash (2 cups/1 whole)
- Zucchini (1 cup)
- Summer squash (1 cup)
- Onions (1 cup)
- Bell peppers - red and green (1 cup of each)
- Quinoa/approved wild rice/grain/pasta (1 cup)
- Basil (1 tbsp.)
- Sea salt (4 tsp.)
- Onion powder (3 tbsp.)
- Fresh ginger (1 tbsp.)
- Oregano (1 tbsp.)
- Cayenne (.25 tsp./optional)

Instructions:

1. Chop the kale—cube the zucchini, peppers, onions, and squash. Mince the ginger.

2. Rinse the soursop leaves, rip them in half, and place them into a large stockpot with spring water (4 cups).
3. Boil leaves for 15-20 minutes with the lid on the pot.
4. Remove leaves from the broth and add the rest of the fixings.
5. Pour in spring water (Add 8 cups for quinoa/maybe more water for grains/rice that absorbs more water)
6. Stir the fixings, replace the lid, and simmer using the medium-temperature setting for 30-45 minutes. (More time possibly needed if not using quinoa.)

Dinner Options

Dr. Sebi's Creamy Kamut "Alkaline" Pasta

Total Time Required: 50 minutes
Yields Provided: 6

Ingredients Needed:
- Spring water - to boil pasta (6-8 cups)
- Kamut Spirathels (12 oz./340.2 g box)
- Grapeseed oil (2 tbsp.)
- Onion powder (1 tsp.)
- Dried tarragon (1 tbsp.)
- Sea salt (1 tsp.)
  The Sauce
- Onion - chopped (half of 1 medium)
- Sliced - baby Bella mushrooms (16 oz./453.6 pkg.)
- Grapeseed oil - divided (2 tbsp.)
- Black pepper & salt (.25 tsp. + .5 tsp. of each)
- Chickpea flour (.25 cup)
- Spring water (2 cups)
- Full-fat unsweetened coconut milk ** (15 oz./425.2 g can)
- Dried tarragon (1 tbsp.)
- Dried basil and oregano (1 tsp. of each)
- Onion powder (2 tsp.)
- Plum/Roma tomatoes - chopped (2-3)

- Packed fresh kale (2 cups)

Instructions:

1. Prepare a big soup pot of water with a pinch of salt. Wait for it to boil.
2. After it's boiling, add the pasta and simmer until it's al dente' (8-10 min.).
3. Once the pasta is ready, drain and add to a bowl. (Keep the pot out as you will need it to make your sauce.)
4. Optionally, season the pasta individually while still warm. You can skip this step if you like. To the warm pasta, add grapeseed oil, dried tarragon, sea salt, and onion powder.
5. Mix - coating your pasta with the seasonings evenly. Set aside to begin making your creamy sauce.
6. Make the sauce. Add grapeseed oil (1 tbsp.) to the same big pot used to boil your pasta. Warm the pot using a med-high temperature setting. To the hot oil - add chopped onions and sliced mushrooms. Simmer, occasionally stirring until the veggies have softened (3-5 min.).
7. Add pepper and salt to your veggies to season and stir. Mix in oil and chickpea flour (1 tbsp. of each).

8. Stir frequently, mixing the flour with the oil and vegetables for no more than one minute.
9. Pour in the spring water, can of coconut milk, tarragon, oregano, basil, onion powder, salt, and black pepper (.5 tsp. each). Simmer with the top 'off' of the pan using the low-temperature setting until the sauce begins to slightly thicken (20 min.).
10. At that time, add in the cooked pasta, tomatoes, and kale. Stir until kale is cooked down (3-5 min.). Remove from heat. Serve immediately.
11. Note ** When using coconut milk, ONLY use unsweetened coconut milk.

Dr. Sebi's Chickpea Loaf

Total Time Required: 1 hour 15 minutes
Yields Provided: 1 loaf

Ingredients Needed:
- Bell peppers (2)
- Onions (1.5 cups)
- Grapeseed oil (2 tbsp.)
- Minced fresh basil (.5 cup)
- Homemade natural granulated onion (2 tbsp. + .5 tsp.)
- Sea salt (1 tsp.)
- Dried sage (.75 tsp.)
- Dried oregano (.5 tsp.)
- Cayenne pepper (.5 tsp.)
- Dried thyme (.25 tsp.)
- Chickpeas, cooked (3 cups)
- Mushrooms (all kinds - except shiitake (1 cup)
- Spelt flour (.5 cup)
- Cayenne pepper & Sea salt (to your liking)

Instructions:
1. Warm the oven to 350° Fahrenheit/177° Celsius.
2. Finely dice the peppers and onions.

3. Sauté the mushrooms with the bell peppers and onion in grapeseed oil over med-high temperature setting (2-3 min.).
4. Stir in minced basil and seasonings. Remove it from heat.
5. Coarsely chop the chickpeas by hand or in a food processor. Stir into the sautéd vegetables. Add spelt flour and mix well.
6. Grease a loaf pan with grapeseed oil. Bake uncovered for 55 to 60 minutes.

<u>Dr. Sebi's Inspired Hot Dogs - Vegan-Friendly</u>

Total Time Required: 1 hour 20 minutes
Yields Provided: 6-10 dogs

Ingredients Needed:
- Garbanzo beans (1 cup)
- Aquafaba (.5 cup)
- Spelt flour (1 cup)
- Green pepper (.33 cup)
- Shallots (.25 cup)
- Onion (.33 cup)
- Ginger (.5 tsp.)
- Smoked sea salt (2 tsp.)
- Onion powder (1 tbsp.)
- Fennel (.5 tsp.)
- Coriander (1 tsp.)
- Dill (.5 tsp.)
- *To Sauté*: Grapeseed oil
  Optional Fixings:
- Crushed red pepper (.5 tsp.)
- Dr. Sebi Inspired Ketchup
- Alkaline Electric Buns*
  Special Tools:
- Hot Dog Mold
- Food Processor
- Taco Rack (if needed)

*If you want to prepare a batch of hot dog buns, follow the buns recipe, then roll out the dough, and bake over a taco rack. If you don't have a rack, you can use tortillas or flatbread.

Instructions:

1. Dice the peppers and onions.
2. Sauté the veggies and garbanzo beans with a tiny bit of oil in a skillet (5 min.).
3. Blend the veggies and the rest of the fixings in the food processor until thoroughly blended.
4. Place the mixture into hot dog mold or roll into a hot dog shape with your hands - wrap in parchment baking paper.
5. Put hot dogs into a steamer over boiling water and steam (30-40 min.).
6. Once the steaming has completed, transfer the hot dogs from the parchment paper or hot dog mold.
7. Brown the hot dogs in a skillet lightly coated with grapeseed oil (5-10 min. using medium heat).
   Serve as desired.

Dr. Sebi's Inspired Meatballs

Total Time Required: 20-25 minutes
Yields Provided: 30-38 meatballs

Ingredients Needed:
- Mushrooms (2 cups)
- Garbanzo bean flour (.5 cup)
- Cooked garbanzo beans (1.5 cups)
- Onions (.5 cup)
- Green peppers (.25 cup)
- Onion powder (1 tbsp.)
- Oregano (2 tsp.)
- Fennel powder (1 tsp.)
- Basil (2 tsp.)
- Sea salt (1 tsp.)
- Ginger powder (.5 tsp.)
- Savory (1 tsp.)
- Dill (1 tsp.)
- Sage (1 tsp.)
- Cayenne powder (.5 tsp.)
- Ground cloves (.5 tsp.)
- Grapeseed oil
- Alkaline tomato sauce (6 cups)
- Food processor

Instructions:

1. Chop the onions and peppers.
2. Toss all of the fixings into the food processor until well blended (1 min.).
3. Add it to a big mixing container. Sift in one cup of flour.
4. Then try to shape it into a ball. Add in more flour if you can't roll into a ball.
5. Roll out the balls and set them aside for cooking.
6. Use the med-high temperature setting.
7. Spritz the skillet with oil and add a few meatballs.
8. Using tongs, flip and cook on each side for about two minutes.
9. Add meatballs to the tomato sauce and allow it to simmer for five minutes.
10. Serve as desired.

Dr. Sebi's Inspired Mushroom "Chicken Tenders"

Total Time Required: varies with the cooking method used
Yields Provided: 6-8 strips from each of the caps

Ingredients Needed:
- Grapeseed oil
- Portobello mushrooms** (2-6)
- Aquafaba/Springwater (1.5 cups)
- Spelt flour (1.5 cups)
- Cayenne powder (1 tsp.)
- Allspice (1 tsp.)
  Spices @ 2 tsp. Each:
- Basil
- Oregano
- Sea salt
- Sage
- Onion powder
- Ginger powder

Instructions:

1. Slice the mushroom caps about ½-inch apart and toss them into a big mixing container. The stems can be chopped to make nuggets.
2. Add the aquafaba, a tiny bit of oil to the container, and ½ of each seasoning.
3. Marinate for about one hour.
4. Whisk the flour with the rest of the seasonings in a big mixing container. Batter the mushrooms.
Baking:
5. Set the oven temperature to 400° Fahrenheit/204° Celsius.
6. Lightly spritz the baking tray with oil. Arrange the mushrooms on the pan.
7. Bake for 15 minutes, and flip - cook until crispy (+ 15 min.).
The Stovetop:
8. Use the med-high temperature setting and add oil to the skillet (3 tbsp.).
9. Sauté the mushrooms on each side until crispy (3-4 min. per side.).
10. **Note: Oyster or white mushrooms can also be used. Adjust the flour and aquafaba to match the number of mushrooms being used as needed.

Dr. Sebi's Mushroom Risotto

Total Time Required: Varies on the method used
Yields Provided: 4-6

Ingredients Needed:
- Grapeseed oil (1 tbsp.)
- Mushrooms (4)
- Sea salt & cayenne pepper (as desired)
- Onion (half of 1)
- Wild rice (2 cups)
- Homemade vegetable broth - made from approved veggies (4 cups)

Instructions:

1. Prepare a big soup pot and heat it using the oil over the medium-temperature setting.
2. Sauté the onions and mushrooms until they're lightly browned, and liquid is evaporated, occasionally stirring (5-7 min.).
3. Stir in rice and simmer for another minute.
4. Mix in the vegetable broth, sea salt, and pepper.
5. Put a lid on the pot and simmer until the rice is tender. Set for the low-temperature setting (2¾ hrs.) or high (1¼ hrs.).

Grilled Zucchini Hummus Wrap

Total Time Required: 15-20 minutes
Yields Provided: 2 tortillas

Ingredients Needed:
- Zucchini (1)
- Plum tomato (1) or cherry tomatoes
- Red onion (¼ of 1)
- Romaine lettuce or wild arugula (1 cup)
- Homemade hummus/mashed garbanzo beans (4 tbsp.)
- Spelt flour tortillas (2)
- Grapeseed oil (1 tbsp.)
- Sea salt & cayenne pepper (as you prefer)

Instructions:

1. Warm a grill or skillet using the medium-temperature setting.
2. Trim the tips from the zucchini. Slice the zucchini, tomatoes, and onion.
3. Toss the zucchini into the oil with a sprinkle of sea salt and cayenne.
4. Arrange the slices of zucchini directly on the grill grate rack to grill for three minutes.
5. Flip them and grill for another two minutes. Set the zucchini aside.

6. Put the tortillas on the grill and cook until grill marks are visible and tortillas are pliable (1 min.).
7. Transfer the tortillas from the grill.

Assemble the wraps as desired. Wrap tightly and enjoy immediately.

Jamaican Jerk Patties - Dr. Sebi Inspired

Total Time Required: 45-60 minutes
Yields Provided: 6-8 empanadas

Ingredients Needed:
- Mushrooms (2 cups)
- Garbanzo beans - cooked (1 cup)
- Butternut squash (1 cup)
- Green pepper (.5 cup)
- Onion (.5 cup)
- Plum tomato (1)
- Raw agave (1 tbsp.)
- Onion powder (1 tbsp.)
- Clove (1 tsp.)
- Thyme (2 tsp.)
- Ginger (1 tsp.)
- Cayenne (.5 tsp.)
- Sea salt (1 tsp.)
- Cloves (.25 tsp.)
  The Crust:
- Spelt flour (1.5 cups)
- Spring water (1 cup)
- Grapeseed oil (1 tbsp.)
- Onion powder (1 tsp.)
- Ginger powder (.125 tsp./a pinch)
- Sea salt (1 tsp.)

- Aquafaba/Garbanzo bean brine/springwater (.25 cup)

Instructions:

1. Chop or mince, and pulse all vegetables (omit the tomato) in the food processor a few times to break down any big chunks.
2. Toss the seasonings, tomato, and vegetables in a mixing container.
3. Make the dough. Whisk the flour with the seasonings and oil in a big mixing container.
4. Add water (¼ cup at a time). Knead until the dough is formed into a ball, adding more flour if too wet.
5. Leave the dough to rest for five to ten minutes. Knead for a couple of minutes.
6. Portion the dough into about eight segments.
7. Warm the oven to reach 350° Fahrenheit/177° Celsius.
8. Roll the prepared dough into balls. Roll each ball into six to seven-inch circles.
9. Load each of the circles with filling (½ cup), brush edges with aquafaba. Fold over and press the dough together with a fork.
10. Gently brush the baking tray using a spritz of oil.
11. Set a timer to bake the patties (25-30 min.).
12. Allow cooling before serving.

Mushroom & Chickpea Burgers

Total Time Required: 20-25 minutes
Yields Provided: 8

Ingredients Needed:
- Green peppers (.5 cup)
- Cayenne (.5 tsp.)
- Red & white onions (.5 cup)
- Cooked chickpeas (2 cups)
- Portobello mushrooms (2)
- Onion powder (2 tsp.)
- Himalayan sea salt (2 tsp.)
- Cilantro (.5 cup)
- Oregano (2 tsp.)
- Garbanzo bean flour (.25 cup)

Instructions:
1. Chop the mushrooms and dice the veggies.
2. Toss all of the prepared fixings into a food processor. Pulse them for about three seconds.
3. Check the consistency of the blend. Mix in additional flour if it appears too moist. Toss it into a mixing container when it's ready.
4. Prepare a skillet using the med-high temperature setting to heat oil.
5. Scoop the burger blend (¼ cup) and add to the skillet.

6. Simmer the burgers for three to five minutes per side before flipping. Be careful when flipping so that the burgers don't crumble.

One-Pot Zucchini Mushroom Pasta

Total Time Required: 40 minutes
Yields Provided: 4-6

Ingredients Needed:
- Approved-grain spaghetti (like spelt or Kamut (1 lb.)
- Cremini mushrooms (1 lb.)
- Zucchini (2)
- Thyme (2 sprigs)
- Sea salt and cayenne pepper (as desired)
- Homemade walnut milk (.25 cup)
- Water

Instructions:

1. Thinly slice the mushrooms. Quarter the zucchini and thinly slice it.
2. Prepare a dutch oven or big stockpot using the med-high temperature-setting, adding spaghetti, mushrooms, zucchini, salt, pepper, and thyme with 4.5 cups of water.
3. Wait for it to boil and lower the temperature setting to simmer with the lid off until the pasta is thoroughly cooked and liquid has reduced (8-10 min.).
4. Stir in homemade walnut milk.
5. Serve immediately.

Plant-Based Quinoa Bowl

Total Time Required: 20 minutes
Yields Provided: 2-3

Ingredients Needed:
- Cooked quinoa (1 cup)
- Approved greens (1 handful)
- Grapeseed oil (1 tbsp.)
- Chopped approved vegetables, such as zucchini, cherry tomatoes, bell pepper, etc. (2 cups)
- Sea salt and cayenne pepper (as desired)

Instructions:

1. Warm a large pan to warm a tablespoon of grapeseed oil.
2. Sauté the chopped vegetables until tender.
3. Mix the vegetables with the cooked quinoa, fresh greens, cayenne, and salt to your liking.

Plant-Based Chickpea Quinoa Burgers

Total Time Required: 45-50 minutes
Yields Provided: 8

Ingredients Needed:
- Onion (¼ of 1)
- Cooked Garbanzo beans/chickpeas (1.5 cups)
- Amaranth - cooked (.25 cup)
- Quinoa (1.5 cups - cooked)
- Fresh (approved) herbs of your choice (2 tbsp.)
- Water (2 tbsp.)
- Cayenne pepper & Sea salt (as desired)
- Vegetables of your choice for serving: cherry tomatoes, green (approved) leaves like wild arugula, watercress or lettuce, etc.
- Raw homemade sesame "tahini" butter (1 tbsp. per patty)

Instructions:

1. Set the oven temperature at 375° Fahrenheit/191° Celsius.
2. Cover a baking tray with a sheet of parchment baking paper.
3. Toss the onion and herbs to finely chop in a food processor.

4. Measure and toss in the chickpeas, quinoa, amaranth, salt, and pepper. Continue to pulse - *don't puree* - it should remain a little chunky.
5. Process until a dough begins to form, adding water while the food processor is running. The mixture should be sticky - not dry or runny.
6. Pop the container of dough in the fridge to chill (15 min.).
7. Once chilled, divide the mixture into eight patties.
8. Arrange them on the tray to bake (20 min.).
9. Flip halfway through and finish with a quick two to three-minute broil so the patties can brown.
10. Serve in an approved-flour bun with homemade raw sesame "tahini" butter and wild arugula, watercress, or lettuce.

Portobello Mushroom Burgers

Total Time Required: 40-45 minutes
Yields Provided: 6

Ingredients Needed:
- Portobello mushroom caps (6 large)
- Avocado oil (4 tbsp.)
- Agave syrup (2 tbsp.)
- Key lime juice (2 tbsp.)
- Extra Veggies: Onions, bell peppers, mushrooms, etc.
- Sea salt & Cayenne pepper (as desired)
- Suggested: 9x13 baking dish

Instructions:

1. Prepare the marinade fixings in a mixing container.
2. Place the mushroom caps (cap side down) in the baking dish. Pour in the marinade and allow the mushrooms to soak for about ½ hour, occasionally brushing the mushrooms' tops.
3. Grill mushrooms beginning with cap side down (for 5-7 min. per side).
4. Continue brushing the mushrooms with the marinade as they cook.

5. Serve on toasted (approved-grain) bread with your favorite toppings or with mixed veggies.

Portobello Tacos

Total Time Required: 30-35 minutes
Yields Provided: 8 tortillas

Ingredients Needed:
- Extra-large portobello mushrooms (2)
- Red bell peppers (2)
- Red onion (half of 1)
- Chopped cherry tomatoes (1 cup)
- Kamut flour tortillas (8 homemade)
- Key lime (1)
- Sea salt and cayenne pepper, or any other approved seasonings (as desired)
- Grapeseed oil (.5 cup)
- Avocado - optional

Instructions:

1. Set the oven temperature to 425° Fahrenheit or 218° Celsius.
2. Slice the portobellos into ½-inch thick wedges.
3. Cut the onion into ½-inch thick rings or half-moons.
4. Slice the bell pepper into ½-inch thick strips.

5. Thoroughly brush the mushrooms with the oil, then use the rest on the red bell pepper, tomatoes, and onions.
6. Dust the portobellos with cayenne pepper, sea salt, and any approved seasoning or spices of your choosing.
7. Roast until portobellos are fork-tender (20 min.).
8. When ready to serve, warm the tortillas, and divide the portobellos and veggies.
9. Serve the portobello tacos with avocado and key lime.

Savory Walnut Meat

Total Time Required: 15 minutes
Yields Provided: 2 cups

Ingredients Needed:
- Walnuts (8 oz. soaked)
- Onions (.5 cup)
- Bell peppers - orange, red & green (.25 cup of each)
- Grapeseed oil (2 tbsp.)
- Onion powder (1 tbsp.)
- Oregano and basil (1 tsp. of each)
- Sea salt (.5 tsp. or as desired)
- Cayenne (.25 tsp.)
- Spring water
- Food processor

Instructions:

1. Soak the walnuts in spring water for several hours or overnight. Discard the used water.
2. Toss the walnuts into the processor and pulse to desired consistency.
3. Add oil to the pan using medium to high heat. Sauté the peppers and onion with seasonings (5-10 min.).

4. Add in spring water (1-2 tbsp. as needed). Sauté to maintain the moisture of the walnut meat.
5. Serve with nachos, pasta, or tacos.

Teff Grain Burgers

Total Time Required: 15-20 minutes
Yields Provided: Varies

Ingredients Needed:
- Cooked tef grain (1.5 cups)
- Garbanzo bean (chickpea) flour (1.5 cups)
- Onion (¼ of 1)
- Bell peppers (.25 cup)
- Oregano + basil (1 tsp. of each)
- Dill (1 tsp.)
- Grapeseed oil (1 tbsp.)
- Sea salt and cayenne pepper (as desired)

Instructions:

1. Dice the peppers and onions.
2. Pour a tablespoon of grapeseed oil into a skillet. Toss in and sauté the peppers and onions until they are tender.
3. Prep a big mixing container and toss the sautéd veggies with the rest of the fixings.
4. Form patties with your hands and cook them in a skillet until crispy (3 min. each side).

Veggie Fajitas Tacos

Total Time Required: 15 minutes
Yields Provided: 6

Ingredients Needed:
- Portobello mushrooms (2-3 large)
- Bell peppers (2)
- Onion (1)
- Juice (half of 1 key lime)
- Grapeseed oil (1 tbsp.)
- Kamut flour/corn-free tortillas/or approved grain (6)
- Approved seasonings - ex. onion powder, habanero, or cayenne pepper (as desired)
- Avocado

Instructions:

1. Use a sharp knife to discard the mushrooms' stems, scoop out the gills if desired, and wipe each of the tops. Cut into slices ($\frac{1}{3}$-inch thick).
2. Thinly slice the onion and peppers.
3. Prepare a big skillet using the medium-temperature setting and add the oil. Toss in the peppers and onions to sauté for about two minutes.

4. Add mushrooms and seasonings. Stir occasionally, cooking until softened (7-8 min.).
5. Heat the tortillas and spoon the fajita mixture into the center of the tortillas.
6. Serve with avocado and a spritz of lime juice.

Zucchini Cakes – Dr. Sebi Inspired

Total Time Required: 20 minutes
Yields Provided: 8-10 cakes

Ingredients Needed:
- Grapeseed oil
- Zucchini (2-3)
- Garbanzo bean flour (.5 cup)
- Onions (.25 cup)
- Green onions (.25 cup)
- Onion powder (1 tsp.)
- Cayenne powder (.5 tsp.)
- Sea salt (1 tsp.)
- Oregano & parsley (1 tsp. of each)
- Hemp milk (.25 cup)
- Food processor with grater/Grater

Instructions:

1. Chop the onions. Shred up the zucchini with a grater.
2. Squeeze the moisture out of zucchini by hand in a strainer.
3. Toss the zucchini, flour, milk, onions, and seasonings in a mixing container.
4. Pour a tiny bit of oil into a frying pan. Heat it using the medium-temperature setting.

5. Scoop the zucchini mixture (⅓ cup) into the skillet. Pat it down with the spatula.

Simmer the cakes for about three to five minutes before flipping on each side.

Chapter 5
<u>Delicious Side Dish Favorites</u>

<u>Dr. Sebi's Alkaline Mushroom Gravy</u>

Total Time Required: 20 minutes
Yields Provided: 1.5 cups

Ingredients Needed:
- Grapeseed oil (2 tbsp.)
- Onion (¼ of 1)
- Mushrooms - any type - except shiitake (1 cup)
- Sea salt & cayenne pepper (1 pinch of each)
- Amaranth or spelt flour (1.5 tbsp.)
- Homemade (approved) vegetable broth (.5 cup)
- Homemade walnut milk (1 cup)
- Finely chopped walnuts (2 tbsp.)
- Fresh thyme (.5 tsp.)

Instructions:

1. Dice the onion and slice the mushrooms.
2. Add grapeseed oil to a large saucepan or cast-iron skillet using the medium-temperature setting.

3. Toss in the onion, mushrooms, salt, and cayenne pepper. Sauté them until the onions are translucent (3-4 min.).
4. Add the flour and whisk to coat—Cook for one minute.
5. Slowly whisk in homemade vegetable broth, salt, cayenne, and milk, starting with ½ cup walnut milk and building up. Cook until thickened, frequently stirring, using the low-temperature setting. Taste and adjust seasonings as needed.
6. Add walnuts and stir to combine. Simmer using the low setting until you're ready to serve, adding more walnut milk as needed if it gets too thick.
7. Serve over plant-based biscuits or bread made with flour from approved grains.

Dr. Sebi's Healthy "Fried-Rice"

Total Time Required: 20 minutes
Yields Provided: 2-3

Ingredients Needed:
- Wild rice or quinoa (1 cup)
- Bell peppers (.5 cup)
- Mushrooms (.5 cup)
- Zucchini (.5 cup)
- Onion (¼ of 1)
- Grapeseed oil (1 tbsp.)
- Sea salt & cayenne pepper (as desired)

Instructions:

1. Cook the quinoa/rice until done (not included in time).
2. Cube the onion, and slice the rest of the veggies.
3. Warm oil in a frying pan to sauté the onions till they're browned.
4. Toss in the remaining vegetables and cook for another five minutes. Make sure they're not too soft.
5. Add the cup of boiled rice, and continue cooking until lightly browned.

Dr. Sebi's Butternut Squash – Hash Browns & Home Fries

Total Time Required: --
Yields Provided: 4-6
Note: Notes: These listed are for preparing one type of hash brown - not both.

Ingredients Needed:
- Butternut squash (half of 1)
- Diced onion (.5 cup)
  Extra Garnishes:
- Onion powder
- Cayenne
- Sea salt
- Grapeseed oil (as needed)

Instructions:

1. You can use any of Dr. Sebi's approved seasonings, but they are optional.
   For Shredded Hash Browns:
2. Chop the ends off the squash and slice away the skin using a vegetable peeler.
3. Slice the squash in half at the neck. Cut the body of the squash in half.
4. Use a spoon to scoop the seeds from the body.

5. Shred the butternut squash with a grater.
6. Lightly coat a skillet with oil and add the shredded onion and squash.
7. Flavor the mixture using sea salt, onion powder, and cayenne to your liking.
8. Let the squash simmer using the med-high temperature setting for about five minutes before flipping, and cook until golden brown.

For Cubed Hash Browns:

9. Chop the ends off the squash and discard the skin with a vegetable peeler.
10. Slice the squash in half at the neck, and slice the body of the squash in half.
11. Discard the seeds from the body.
12. Chop the butternut squash into ½-inch squares and dice ½ of an onion.
13. Lightly coat the pan using oil. Add your chopped squash and onion with spices to your liking.
14. Sauté the squash on medium-high heat until brown (8-10 min.).

Bread Options

<u>Dr. Sebi's Inspired Buns</u>

Total Time Required: ½ hours
Yields Provided: 4-6

Ingredients Needed:
- Grapeseed oil (2 tsp.)
- Spelt Flour (2.25-2.5 cups)
- Sparkling spring water (.25 cup)
- Hemp/Walnut milk (.5 cup)
- Aquafaba (.25 cup)
- Agave (1 tbsp.)
- Sea salt (1.5 tsp.)
- Onion powder (1 tbsp.)
- Oregano/basil (1 tsp.)
- Sea Moss Gel (1 tsp./optional)
- Sesame seeds (optional)
- Mixer with a dough hook*
- *You can also process and knead by hand.
- Baking sheet

Instructions:

1. Toss all of the dry fixings into the mixing bowl. Mix until blended.
2. Add in the remainder of the fixings. Blend for one minute using the low-speed setting.

Knead the dough at medium speed for five minutes or by hand (8-10 min. if).

3. Arrange a layer of parchment baking paper on a baking tray. Spritz or brush the paper with a drizzle of oil.
4. Divide the dough into separate parts (4-6), roll in your hands. Shape the dough and place it on the tray.
5. Lightly brush each of the buns with oil and garnish with a sprinkle of sesame seeds.
6. Cover the tray using a piece of plastic wrap. Let the buns rest for ½ hour.
7. Warm the oven to reach 350° Fahrenheit/177° Celsius.
8. Bake the bread for 25-30 minutes.
9. Allow buns to cool, carefully cut them in half, and serve.

<u>Dr. Sebi's Inspired Spelt & Rye Bread</u>

Total Time Required: 1.75-2 hours
Yields Provided: 1 loaf

Ingredients Needed:
- Rye & spelt flour (2 cups of each type)
- Dr. Sebi Bromide Plus Powder (.5 tsp.) or Sea Moss* (2 tbsp.)
- Sea salt (1 tsp.)
- Hemp Milk (2 cups)
- Agave (2 tbsp.)
- Optional: Sesame seeds
- Mixer with a dough hook
- Loaf pan (1)

Instructions:

1. Set the oven to 350° F/177° C.
2. Thoroughly whisk or sift the flour into a mixing container.
3. Pour dry fixings into a mixer bowl and start the mixer using the low-speed setting.
4. Add the milk - while mixing, scraping the flour off the side and bottom when needed.
5. Add the agave while the mixer is off, and then mix for about five minutes.
6. With the mixer going, "grease & flour" a loaf pan by lightly coating it with oil and flour.

Scoop the dough into the loaf pan and even it out. Add more flour to the top of your cooking utensil sticks.

7. Lightly brush oil over the top of the bread. Sprinkle it using sesame seeds.
8. Place the bread in the oven for one hour.
9. Transfer it to a cooling rack until cool (20 min.).
10. If you choose to use the sea moss as a gel, it might make the batter a tiny bit stickier.

Fantastic Quinoa Bread

Total Time Required: 2¼ hours
Yields Provided: 1 loaf

Ingredients Needed:
- Whole uncooked quinoa seed (300 g/10.5 oz./1.75 cups)
- Water (.5 cup)
- Grapeseed oil (60 ml/2 fl oz./.25 cup)
- Sea salt (.5 tsp.)
- Key lime - juiced (half of 1)

Instructions:

1. The day before, soak quinoa in a container of cold water in the fridge.
2. Warm the oven to reach 320° Fahrenheit/160° Celsius.
3. Prepare a loaf pan with a sheet of parchment baking paper (bottom and sides).
4. Drain the quinoa and thoroughly rinse it through a sieve. Scoop the quinoa into a food processor.
5. Measure and mix in sea salt, oil, water (½ cup), and key lime juice.
6. Mix in a food processor for three minutes.
7. Spoon the mixture into the prepared pan.

8. Set a timer to bake the bread for 1½ hours until it's firm to the touch and bounce back when pressed with your fingers.
9. Transfer the pan to the countertop/stovetop to cool for ½ hour in the pan.
10. The bread should be slightly moist in the middle and crisp on the outside.
11. Transfer it to a cooling rack until it's entirely cooled before eating.

Veggies

<u>Alkaline Electric Burro Mashed "Potatoes"</u>

Total Time Required: 35 minutes
Yields Provided: 4-6

Ingredients Needed:
- Green burro bananas (6-8)** or Cooked garbanzo beans (2 cups)
- Walnut/hemp milk (1 cup)
- Onion powder (2 tsp.)
- Sea salt (2 tsp.)
- Green onions (.25 cup)

Instructions:
1. Chop off each burro's ends, cut into the skin on each side, then remove the skin and add to a food processor.
2. Pour in the milk and seasonings. Blend for one to two minutes, adding spring water if the blend needs thinning.
3. Dice and add the green onions into a saucepan and cook on a medium-temperature setting.
4. Cook for 25-30 minutes while constantly stirring, adding more water as it gets too thick.

5. Serve with some delicious gravy!
6. Note:** Be sure the skin is still green; otherwise, it will taste sweet if the skin turns yellow. You will acquire a slight taste of banana when using burros.

Basil Pesto "Zoodles"

Total Time Required: 15-20 minutes
Yields Provided: 6-8

Ingredients Needed:
- Zucchini (1 lb.)
- Grapeseed oil (1 tbsp.)
- Ripe avocado (1)
- Packed basil leaves (.5 cup)
- Walnuts (.25 cup)
- Olive oil (.25 cup)
- Sea salt (.5 tsp.)
- Cayenne pepper (.25 tsp.)
- Cherry tomatoes (1 cup)
- Juice (1 key lime)

Instructions:

1. Slice the zucchini into small strips.
2. Prepare the zoodles by sautéing the zucchini noodles with grapeseed oil until slightly tender but still crunchy.
3. Toss the remainder of the fixings in a blender and work it into a creamy, thick paste.
4. Add to the drained pasta and toss and combine. If the sauce is too thick, add a tiny bit of water.

5. Serve and enjoy it with cherry tomato halves and decorate with shredded desiccated coconut as "cheese."

Creamy Citrus Greens

Total Time Required: 10-15 minutes
Yields Provided: 4

Ingredients Needed:
- Favorite approved greens - kale, dandelion, turnip greens, amaranth, purslane (5 oz./150 g)
- Cubed approved green vegetables - chayote, zucchini, green bell pepper (5 oz./150 g)
- To Sauté: Oil - hemp seed - grapeseed or avocado oil
- Freshly squeezed orange juice (3 fl oz./90 ml)
- Juice (half of 1 lime)
- Onion (1 small)
- Optional: Dates (1-2 soaked)
- Tahini (1-2 tbsp.)
- Sea salt & cayenne pepper (as desired)

Instructions:

1. Steam the leafy greens until they change color slightly and become softer.
2. Simmer the cubed green vegetables in water or a tiny bit of oil.

3. Make the dressing by blending the rest of the fixings until smooth. Add more tahini to thicken.
4. Optionally, sweeten with soaked dates.
5. Liberally drizzle the dressing over the greens with a pinch more cayenne as desired.

Dr. Sebi's Inspired "Potato" Salad

Total Time Required: 45-50 minutes
Yields Provided: 4

Ingredients Needed:
- Cooked garbanzo beans (2 cups) or Green bananas (4)*
- Brazil nuts - soaked overnight (1 cup)
- Spring water - warm is preferred (1 cup)
- Green peppers (.25 cup)
- Onions (.25 cup)
- Lime juice (1-1.5 tbsp.)
- Avocado oil (2 tsp.)
- Sea salt (1 tsp.)
- Onion powder (1 tsp.)
- Dill (1 tsp.)
- Ginger powder (.5 tsp.)
- Optional: Sea Moss Gel (.5 tsp.)
- Cayenne powder (1 pinch)
- Optional Topping: Annatto/Achiote Powder
  *Steps 1, 4, & 5 can be left out of the recipe steps if using garbanzo beans.

Instructions:

1. Cut bananas in half, scrape off the skin, and chop into cubes.

2. Load the blender. Add in the seasonings, nuts, oil, spring water (½ cup), and lime juice. Mix for one minute.
3. Add spring water (¼ cup) and sea moss gel. Blend until smooth and store it in the fridge. (Mix in more water if it needs thinning.)
4. Pour water in a pan and wait for it to boil. Toss in and stir the bananas until translucent (2-4 min.).
5. Strain the bananas into a mixing container.
6. Dice/chop and add the green peppers, onions, and nut mixture to the bowl and thoroughly mix.
7. Store in the fridge until chilled (½ hour).

Spicy Sesame Squash

Total Time Required: 20-25 minutes
Yields Provided: 4

Ingredients Needed:
- Squash (1 medium)
- Sesame oil (2 tbsp.)
- Sea salt and cayenne pepper (1 pinch)
- Sesame seeds (4 tbsp.)

Instructions:
1. Cut the squash into small cubes of approximately 1-cm or ⅓ inch.
2. Sprinkle them using a pinch of cayenne and salt.
3. Sauté using the low-temperature setting in sesame oil until golden brown (15 min.).
4. Toast the sesame seeds in a hot 'dry' frying pan until they begin popping.
5. Transfer the pan to a cool burner and sprinkle seeds over the squash before serving.

Stewed Okra & Tomatoes

Total Time Required: 40-45 minutes
Yields Provided: 4

Ingredients Needed:
- Fresh okra (2 cups)
- Cherry tomatoes (1 cup)
- Onion (1 medium)
- Avocado oil (1 tbsp.)
- Fresh spring water (.5 cup)
- Cayenne pepper & sea salt (as desired)

Instructions:

1. Peel and dice the onion and dice the cherry tomatoes.
2. Warm the oil in a frying pan and toss in the onion. Sauté until the onion is translucent.
3. Chop and toss in the okra and spring water. Simmer it for ten minutes using the low-temperature setting.
4. Fold in the tomatoes and simmer until the okra is cooked through (20 min.).
5. Sprinkle it with pepper and sea salt as desired to serve.

Vegetable Alfredo - Dr. Sebi Style

Total Time Required: 15-20 minutes
Yields Provided: 4-6

Ingredients Needed:
- Spelt Tortiglioni Pasta (10 oz./280 g bag)
- Brazil nut cheese sauce
- Mushrooms (1 container)
- Summer & zucchini squash (1 of each)
- Bell peppers - red & orange (1 of each)
- Onion (1)
  As Desired:
- Cayenne
- Basil
- Onion powder
- Oregano
- Sea salt
- Grapeseed oil

Instructions:

1. Boil pasta according to directions (8-10 min.). Drain it into a colander.
2. Chop the veggies.
3. Pour oil into the skillet. Toss in some of each vegetable.
4. Add 1 tsp. of herbs and seasonings.

5. Lightly sauté the vegetables for about two minutes using the medium-temperature setting.
6. Mix in the pasta and cheese sauce.
7. Toss and sauté them for about one minute.
8. Serve with your favorite toppings.

<u>Vegetable Quinoa - Dr. Sebi Style</u>

Total Time Required: 20 minutes
Yields Provided: 6-8

Ingredients Needed:
- Cooked quinoa (4 cups)
- Zucchini (1 cup)
- Red - yellow & green bell peppers (.25 cup of each)
- Spring water (.5 cup)
- Red onion (.5 cup)
- Roma/Plum tomato (1)
- Grapeseed/Olive oil (2 tbsp./optional)
- Onion powder (1 tbsp.)
- Oregano and basil (1 tsp. each)
- Cayenne powder (.5 tsp.)
- Sea salt (2 tsp.)

Instructions:
1. Dice the bell peppers, onions, and tomatoes. Chop the zucchini.
2. Pour oil into a big frying pan and heat using the med-high temperature setting.
3. Sauté the vegetables and seasonings for five to ten minutes.
4. Stir in the quinoa and water. Continue to simmer another five minutes to serve.

Chapter 6
Snacks & Appetizer Favorites

Alkaline-Electric Apple Bake

Total Time Required: 1 hour 15 minutes
Yields Provided: 4

Ingredients Needed:
- Gala or Honeycrisp apples (3 - 4)
- Agave syrup (3 tbsp.)
- Chopped walnuts (1 tbsp.)
- Cloves (1 pinch)

Instructions:

1. Warm the oven to 350° Fahrenheit/177° Celsius.
2. Thinly slice the apples. Toss them into a big mixing container with a drizzle of agave syrup. Stir well to coat.
3. Toss the cloves and walnuts. Sprinkle over the apples, stirring while sprinkling. Let the flavors meld for about five minutes to produce the juices.
4. Arrange the sliced apples into a casserole dish. Bake them for 15 minutes.

5. Cover with foil. Bake till the apples are bubbly (35-40 min.).
6. Serve when ready.

Baked Avocado with Salsa & Sides

Total Time Required: 45 minutes
Yields Provided: 4

Ingredients Needed:
- Avocados (2 large)
- Chopped fresh basil (1 oz.) or Dried (1 tsp.)
- Fresh plum tomatoes (4) or Cherry tomatoes (30)
- Onions (4 small)
- Cayenne pepper (1 pinch)

Instructions:

1. Warm the oven to reach 302° Fahrenheit/150° Celsius.
2. Chop the tomatoes and onions into small pieces, dusting with pepper and salt.
3. Slice the avocados in half and discard the stone.
4. Fill the avocado halves with the tomato mixture.
5. Bake for ½ hour.
6. Serve as desired.

Dr. Sebi Inspired Applesauce

Total Time Required: 10 minutes
Yields Provided: 4

Ingredients Needed:
- Apples (3 cups)
- Lime juice (1 tsp.)
- Cloves (125 tsp./1 pinch)
- Agave (3 tbsp.)
- Sea salt (.125 tsp./1 pinch)
- Strawberries* (.5 cup/optional)
- Sea moss gel (1 tsp./optional)
- Spring water (optional)

Instructions:

1. Peel, chop, and toss the apples into a blender with the agave, cloves, salt, and lime juice.
2. Reach the desired consistency using a blender. Pulse in the berries until well blended. (Mix in one tablespoon of spring water at a time as needed)
3. Serve and save the leftovers in the fridge for later.

Dr. Sebi Inspired Candied Walnuts & Strawberry Dressing

Total Time Required: 15 minutes
Yields Provided: 2 to 4 - varies upon how it's used

Ingredients Needed:
The Walnuts:
- Walnuts (.5 cup)
- Agave nectar - raw (1 tbsp.)
- Sea salt (.25 cup)

The Dressing:
- Sliced strawberries (.5 cup)
- Shallots (2 tbsp.)
- Optional: Grapeseed - olive or avocado oils (.5 cup)
- Raw agave nectar (2 tsp.)
- Lime juice (1.5 tsp.)
- Onion powder (1 tsp.)
- Ginger (half of 1)
- Dill (.25 tsp.)
- Sea salt (.25 tsp.)

Instructions:

1. Warm the oven to reach at 325° Fahrenheit/163° Celsius.

2. Coat the walnuts with agave and salt.
3. Place on a cookie tray lined with parchment baking paper.
4. Bake for 8-10 min.
5. Cool and enjoy as a snack or on a salad.
6. Toss the dressing fixings in a cup and blend for about ½ minute to serve.

<u>Dr. Sebi Inspired Spelt & Rye Crackers</u>

Total Time Required: 20-25 minutes/batch
Yields Provided: 50 crackers - according to size cooked

Ingredients Needed:
- Spelt flour (1-1.25 cups)
- Rye flour (.5 cup)
- Grapeseed oil (2 tbsp.)
- Sesame seeds (2 tsp.)
- Spring water (.75 cup)
- Sea salt (1 tsp.)
- Agave (1 tsp.)
- Herb of choice (1 pinch)

Instructions:

1. Start by only using ¾ cup of spelt flour. (Mix in the remaining 1/3 cup of spelt till you've mixed the other fixings).
2. Toss all of the fixings into a mixing container to make the dough.
3. Warm the oven to 350° Fahrenheit/177° Celsius.
4. Prepare the countertop or cutting board to roll the dough and cover it using a layer of parchment baking paper.

5. Pour a tiny bit of oil onto the paper. Roll the dough ball using a rolling pin. Add more flour as needed if the dough is sticking to the rolling pin.
6. Use your shape cutter to cut circles in the dough. You can also place the dough on the baking sheet and use a pizza cutter. Remove the dough surrounding the circles and make it into a ball to reshape.
7. Once on the baking sheet, poke tiny holes in the dough using a toothpick to help them cook evenly on both sides.
8. Brush the crackers gently with oil and sprinkle them using a sprinkle of salt.
9. Bake in the oven for 10-15 minutes and cool to serve.

Dr. Sebi's No-Bake Energy Balls

Total Time Required: 40 minutes
Yields Provided: Vary

Ingredients Needed:
- Raspberries (.75 cup)
- Dates (10)
- Walnuts (1 cup)
- Shredded soft-jelly coconut meat (2 ⅔ cups)
- Sea salt (1 pinch)

Instructions:

1. Toss each of the fixings into a blender/food processor. Mix it until they're fully incorporated.
2. Use moist hands to shape the mixture into balls.
3. Arrange them on a baking sheet and place them in the freezer for 20-30 minutes. Serve as desired when ready.

Dr. Sebi's Inspired Quiche

Total Time Required: 1 hour 15 minutes
Yields Provided: 6

Ingredients Needed:
The Crust:
- Spring water (1 cup)
- Spelt flour/garbanzo bean flour (1 cup)
- Oregano (1 tsp.)
- Onion powder (1 tsp.)
- Basil (1 tsp.)
- Sea salt (1 tsp.)
The Filling:
- Garbanzo bean flour (1 cup)
- Kale (1 cup)
- Mushrooms - sliced (2 cups)
- Brazil nut cheese (1 cup)
- Hemp milk/or another approved nut milk (.75 cup)
- Aquafaba (.75 cup)
- Onions -white and red (.5 cup)
- Bell peppers - green and yellow (.5 cup)
- Alkaline "garlic sauce" (see recipe above for 1 tbsp.)
- Sea Moss gel (1 tbsp./optional - see recipe)
- Oregano (1 tsp.)
- Onion powder (1 tbsp.)

- Basil (1 tsp.)
- Sea salt (1 tsp.)
- Cayenne powder (.25 tsp.)
- Grapeseed oil (as needed)

Instructions:

1. Blend the seasonings and flour for the crust.
2. Mix in water - about ¼ cup at a time - until the dough can be formed into a ball, adjusting flour as needed.
3. Dust a cutting board and roll the dough to fit into a pie platter.
4. Lightly coat the pie pan with oil, then fit dough into the pan and trim off the edges.
5. Combine quiche mixture (flour, milk, aquafaba, sea moss gel, "garlic" sauce, and seasonings) into a blender. Pulse until incorporated.
6. Set the oven temperature setting to reach 350° Fahrenheit/177° Celsius.
7. Chop the kale. Toss the onions, mushrooms peppers, and kale in a large mixing container.
8. Add the mixed veggies into the pan, cover with the nut cheese, and pour in quiche mixture.
9. Lay foil over the pie pan.
10. Bake it for 55-65 minutes.

11. Remove foil for the last ten minutes of cooking.
12. Cool the quiche before slicing it to serve.

<u>Dr. Sebi's Inspired Roasted Tomato Sauce</u>

Total Time Required: 1 hour 10 minutes
Yields Provided: 6 cups

Ingredients Needed:
- Roma tomatoes (18)
- Red bell pepper (half of 1)
- Sweet onion (half of 1)
- Red onion (half of 1)
- Medium shallot (1)
- Grapeseed oil (1/8 cup)
- Sea salt (3 tsp.)
- Agave (1 tbsp.)
- Oregano (2 tsp.)
- Cayenne powder (1/8 tsp.)
- Basil (3 tsp.)
- Onion powder (2 tsp.)
- Pot – at least 4-Quart

Instructions:

1. Warm the oven temperature setting to 400° Fahrenheit/204° Celsius.
2. Cut all vegetables in half and place them in a mixing container.
3. Add grapeseed oil with one teaspoon each of sea salt and basil.

4. Toss vegetables in the mixture until they are fully coated.
5. Place all vegetables cut side down on a baking tray lined with parchment baking paper.
6. Roast in the oven for ½ hour, turning the cookie sheet halfway through cooking time.
7. Place roasted vegetables into the blender and mix on high speed until smooth.
8. Pour into the pot along with all remaining ingredients and continue cooking on a low-temperature setting for 20 minutes.

Dr. Sebi's Raw Blueberry Energy Balls

Total Time Required: varies - .5-2 hours
Yields Provided: varies

Ingredients Needed:
- Blueberries or another approved fruit (.5 cup)
- Shredded soft-jelly coconut (2 cups)
- Walnuts or Brazil nuts (.5 cup)
- Dried dates (.5 cup)
- Date sugar (1 tsp.)
- Agave syrup (1 tbsp.)
- Sea salt (1 pinch)

Instructions:

1. Prep the nuts in a food processor or high-speed blender until you get a fine powder.
2. Add the dried dates, date sugar, and blueberries. Slowly, pour the agave syrup until you have a soft paste.
3. Chill mixture for 30 minutes to two hours.
4. Roll into one tablespoon balls, and roll them in more shredded coconut if you like.
5. It will stay tasty in the fridge for seven days or the freezer for up to three months.

<u>Falafel with Red Pepper & Raspberry Coulis</u>

Total Time Required: Varies + 12 hours soaking time
Yields Provided: 4

Ingredients Needed:
- Dried garbanzo beans (3.5 oz./100 g)
- White onion (half of 1 large)
- Sweeter onions of choice (2 small)
- Juice (½ a key lime)
- Sea salt (.25 tsp.)
- Fresh herbs - basil, oregano, thyme (2 oz. - 3 oz./30 g - 50 g)
- Oil to sauté (grapeseed, sesame seed, hemp seed, or avocado oil)
  Sauce Ingredients:
- Red pepper (1)
- Onion (½ of 1 medium)
- Oil for sautéing (grapeseed, sesame seed, hemp seed, or avocado oil)
- Fresh or frozen raspberries (or another 'tart' tasting berry (2 oz./50 g)
- Dates (2 or 3)
- Warm spring water (1.5 fl oz./50 ml)

Instructions:

1. *Preparation*: Soak the dried beans overnight (12 hours) in spring water.
2. *The Falafel*: Put the soaked garbanzo, onion, sea salt, coriander, and lime in a food processor.
3. Blend until you have a fine - yet rough texture.
4. Place mixture in the refrigerator for one hour until firm to make shaping them much more manageable.
5. Shape the falafel into small patties (2-3-cm diameter, 0.5 to 1-cm high or ¾-inch-1-inch diameter, ¼ inch to ⅓-inch high)
6. Sauté in a frying pan using the medium temperature setting until golden brown (3-5 min. per side).
7. *The Sauce*: Put dates in the warm water and soak for 15 minutes.
8. Sauté the onions and red pepper in a tiny bit of oil, in a saucepan, until softened.
9. Add the raspberries and soaked dates (removing the stone).
10. Add the water from the soaked dates. Bring gently to boil for two minutes.
11. Transfer the pan to the countertop and mix until it's creamy smooth.
12. Sieve the sauce through a tea strainer for a super-smooth and seed-free option.

"Heart-Friendly" Salsa

Total Time Required: 5-10 minutes
Yields Provided: 4-6

Ingredients Needed:
- Fresh blueberries (1 cup)
- Strawberries (5 medium)
- Sea salt (1 pinch)
- Grapeseed oil (2 tbsp.)
- Onion (¼ of 1 red)
- Bell pepper - green (.33 or 1/3 cup)
- Avocado (½ of 1)
- Juice (2 key limes)

Instructions:
1. Thoroughly rinse the berries. Chop the onion, pepper, and avocado—Juice the limes.
2. Toss the blueberries, strawberries, onion, key lime zest, key lime juice, and green bell pepper in a food processor or blender. Pulse it five or six times.
3. Taste test and season as desired using a bit of salt and cayenne pepper.
4. Scrape the salsa into a bowl and fold in chopped avocado.

Magic Green Falafels

Total Time Required: approx. 2 hrs.
Yields Provided: Varies upon sizes made.

Ingredients Needed:
- Dry garbanzo beans/chickpeas (2 cups)
- Onion (1 large)
- Bell pepper - red (.33 or 1/3 cup)
- Sea salt (1 tsp.)
- Fresh basil (.66 or 2/3 cup)
- Oregano (.25 tsp.)
- Fresh dill (.5 cup)
- Garbanzo bean flour (.5 cup)
- Grapeseed or avocado oil for frying

Instructions:

1. Chop the onion and pepper.
2. Make the falafels by cooking the chickpeas until softened. Drain and thoroughly rinse the beans and toss them into a food processor along with all the rest of the fixings; red bell pepper, onion, fresh herbs, oregano, sea salt, and flour.
3. Pulse until each of the fixings are finely chopped - producing a coarse meal. Scrape the container and pulse again until the

texture is a fine meal. Taste and adjust the seasonings as needed.

4. Scoop the mixture into a big mixing container. Shape it into small balls or thick discs. Arrange them on a plate lined with a layer of parchment baking paper. Chill in the fridge for at least one hour.
5. Fill a large skillet with oil (a depth of about one inch). Warm it using the medium-temperature setting (5-7 min.).
6. Once the oil is heated, fry the falafels for two to three minutes per side.
7. Serve as desired.

Mango Salsa Specialty

Total Time Required: 10-15 minutes
Yields Provided: 3 cups

Ingredients Needed:
- Roma tomatoes (6)
- Tomatillo (1)
- Red onions (.5 cup)
- Green peppers (.25 cup)
- Mango (.5 cup)
- Lime juice (half of 1 lime)
- Cilantro (.5 cup)
- Onion powder (1 tsp.)
- Cayenne powder (.5 tsp.)
- Sea salt (1 tsp.)

Instructions:

1. Chop the mango and other veggies as desired.
2. Add all of the fixings, except the mango, into a food processor.
3. Pulse for about ten seconds.
4. Scrape off the sides and add mango.
5. Pulse until the mango is thoroughly mixed with the salsa.

Margarita Pizza – Dr. Sebi Inspired

Total Time Required: 40-45 minutes + 2 hours to overnight soaking
Yields Provided: 4-6

Ingredients Needed:
The Crust:
- Spelt flour (1.5 cups)
- Onion powder (.5 tsp.)
- Spring water (1 cup)
- Basil (.5 tsp.)
- Oregano (.5 tsp.)
- Sea salt (.5 tsp.)

The Cheese:
- Spring water (.5 cup)
- Brazil nuts (1 cup - soaked/2 hrs. using hot water)
- Hemp milk/your preference of nut milk (.25 cup)
- Sea Moss Gel (1 tsp./optional)
- Lime juice (1 tsp.)
- Onion powder (.5 tsp.)
- Sea salt (.25 tsp.)
- Oregano (.5 tsp.)
- Basil (.5 tsp.)

The Toppings:
- Red onion

- Plum tomatoes
- Alkaline "Garlic" Sauce (see recipe)
- Fresh basil

Instructions:

1. Set the oven temperature to 350° Fahrenheit/177° Celsius.
2. Lightly spritz the baking pan with a spritz of oil.
3. Whisk the flour and seasonings in a mixing container.
4. Stir in spring water (½ cup), continuing to add water until the dough is worked into a ball.
5. On a floured surface, roll the dough out by rolling in one direction, flipping and turning after every few rolls.
6. Fit the dough into a baking sheet, poking tiny holes with a fork. Bake for 10-15 minutes.
7. Transfer it to the countertop.
8. Adjust the temperature setting to 425° Fahrenheit/218° Celsius. Move the rack to the lowest setting.
9. Add all cheese fixings to a blender, and mix until smooth (1-2 min.).
10. Once the crust is done, coat the pizza with garlic sauce, cheese.

11. Slice and add the desired toppings. Top off with more garlic sauce and cheese if desired.
12. Set a timer to bake it for 10-15 minutes and serve.

Nori-Burritos

Total Time Required: 10-15 minutes
Yields Provided: 4 sheets

Ingredients Needed:
- Avocado (1 ripe)
- Cucumber - seeded (1 lb./450 g)
- Mango, ripe (half of 1)
- Nori seaweed (4 sheets)
- Zucchini (1 small)
- Amaranth or dandelion greens (1 handful)
- Sprouted hemp seeds (1 handful)
- Tahini (1 tbsp.)
- Sesame seeds (as desired)

Instructions:

1. Arrange a Nori sheet on a cutting board or other working surface with its shiny side facing down.
2. Arrange all the ingredients on the nori sheet, leaving an inch wide margin of uncovered nori to the right.
3. Using both hands, fold the sheet of nori from the edge closest to you, rolling it up and over the fillings.

4. Cut in thick slices and sprinkle with sesame seeds.
5. This would pair perfectly with a *Wakame Salad*.

Hummus

Avocado - Apple & Walnut Hummus

Total Time Required: 1.5 hours
Yields Provided: 4

Ingredients Needed:
- Dried garbanzo beans (3.5 oz./100 g)
- Ripe avocado (1 large)
- Tahini (ground sesame seeds (2 tbsp.)
- Small onions (2)
- Key limes (2 juiced)
- Sea salt (.5 tsp.)
- Springwater (1.5 fl oz./50ml)
- Cayenne or African bird pepper (1 pinch)
- Apple (¼ of 1)
- Walnuts (4)
- Cucumber (1 sliced diagonally) or any approved veggie you'd like to dip)

Instructions:

1. Soak dry garbanzo beans overnight (12 hours minimum) in spring water.
2. Alternatively, unsoaked beans can be cooked in a pressure cooker (45 min.).

3. Cook soaked garbanzo beans in a pan of boiling water (medium heat for ½ hour) until soft.
4. Finely chop the onion—Juice the lime and dice the apple.
5. Blend the cooked garbanzo, avocado, tahini, onion, lime, salt, and water (slowly adding water as needed).
6. Sprinkle chopped apple, walnuts, and a pinch of cayenne pepper and serve with sliced cucumber.

Classic Homemade Hummus

Total Time Required: 5 minutes

Ingredients Needed:
- Cooked chickpeas (1 cup)
- Key lime juice (2 tbsp.)
- Homemade tahini butter (.33 cup)
- Olive oil (2 tbsp.)
- Sea salt (as desired)
- Onion powder (1 dash)

Instructions:

1. Toss the fixings into the blender/processor.
2. Set it to the high function, blend, and serve.

Irresistible Red Pepper Hummus

Total Time Required: 25 minutes
Yields Provided: 4-6

Ingredients Needed:
- Olive oil (2 tbsp.)
- Red bell pepper (1)
- Cooked chickpeas (garbanzo beans (1 cup)
- Key lime juice (2 tbsp.)
- Homemade tahini (3 tbsp.)
- Sea salt & Cayenne pepper (as desired)

Instructions:

1. Place the red bell pepper on the stove broiler and roast until the skin has become charred. Scoop it into a plastic bag and wait until they are cool enough to handle (10-15 min.). Remove the skin.
2. Combine the tahini and lime juice in the mixing bowl of a food processor.
3. Process them for one minute, scraping the bottom and sides.
4. Then process it for another ½ minute to help "whip" or "cream" the tahini, making the hummus creamy.
5. Mix in the chickpeas, oil, sea salt, and cayenne pepper. Process for ½ minute,

scraping the sides and bottom, and process for another 30 seconds or until well blended.

6. This red pepper chickpea hummus would be a fantastic topping for a *Plant-Based Quinoa Bowl*.

Condiments

<u>Dr. Sebi's Inspired BBQ Sauce</u>

Total Time Required: 25 minutes + waiting time
Yields Provided: 8-10 oz. sauce

Ingredients Needed:
- Plum tomatoes (6)
- Agave (2 tbsp.)
- Date sugar (.25 cup)
- White onions (.25 cup)
- Regular/Smoked sea salt (2 tsp.)
- Ground ginger (.5 tsp.)
- Onion powder (2 tsp.)
- Cloves (1/8 tsp.)
- Cayenne powder (.25 tsp.)

Instructions:

1. Chop the onions.
2. Add all of the fixings, except date sugar, into a blender and mix until it's creamy smooth.
3. Prepare a saucepan using the med-high temperature setting to blend the date sugar and the rest of the fixings.

4. Once boiling, adjust the temperature to simmer. Place a top on the pot a for 15 minutes, stirring occasionally (15 min.).
5. Use a stick blender to make the sauce creamier.
6. Continue simmering using the lowest temperature setting to cook-down the water (10 min.). Let it cook and thicken further before serving.
7. The longer you wait, the tastier it will be for your favorite portion!

Dr. Sebi's Inspired "Garlic" Sauce

Total Time Required: 1 hour 10 minutes
Yields Provided: 1 cup

Ingredients Needed:
- Grapeseed oil (1 cup)
- Shallots (.25 cup)
- Onion powder (1 tbsp.)
- Ginger (.5 tsp.)
- Sea salt (.25 tsp.)
- Dill (.25 tsp.)
- Stick blender (optional)

Instructions:

1. Mince and add oil, the shallots, and seasonings into a glass jar and shake well.*
2. Allow setting at least one hour before using and store in the refrigerator.
3. *If you combine the fixings using a stick mixer, you can use the sauce right away.

Chapter 7
<u>Dessert Favorites</u>

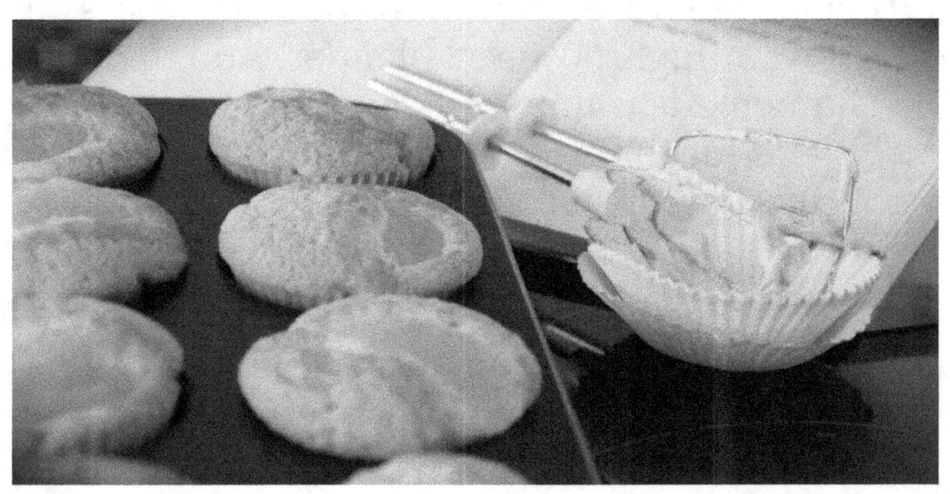

<u>Alkaline-Electric Banana-Mango Ice Cream</u>

Total Time Required: 5 minutes
Yields Provided: 2-4

Ingredients Needed:
- Ripe mangoes (2)
- Burro bananas (2)
- Homemade walnut milk (3 tbsp.)
- Optional: Agave syrup/date sugar

Instructions:

1. Peel and cut the mangoes into cubes. Peel the burro bananas as well, and slice.
2. Put the banana pieces and mango in a baking tray lined with parchment paper. Freeze.
3. Place the frozen fruit into the food processor bowl or high-powered blender. Add the homemade walnut milk and the sweetener.
4. Blend for three to four minutes.
5. Stir and serve as desired.

Alkaline-Electric Banana-Strawberry-Avocado Ice Cream

Total Time Required: 5-6 minutes + freezing time (4-6 hours)
Yields Provided: 1 quart

Ingredients Needed:
- Frozen baby bananas (5)
- Frozen strawberries (1 cup)
- Avocado (half of 1)
- Hemp/your favorite nut milk (.25 cup)
- Agave (1 tbsp.)

Instructions:

1. Toss each of the fixings into a blender and thoroughly mix.
2. Taste and add more agave as desired or milk if it's too thick.
3. Place in an air-tight container and freeze until firm.
4. Scoop out ice cream and serve
5. **Notes: Using frozen fruits isn't essential, but it does help the ice cream to set faster.
6. If it is too hard to scoop, let it soften for a few minutes. If frozen overnight, it might need to sit out for 20 minutes to ½ hour.

<u>Alkaline Electric Spelt Meal Raisin Cookies</u>

Total Time Required: 25-30 minutes/batch
Yields Provided: vary

Ingredients Needed:
- Spelt flour (3 cups)
- Dates - pitted (1.5 cups)
- Homemade applesauce/pureed apple (.66 or 2/3 cup)
- Agave syrup (.33 cup)
- Grapeseed oil (.33 cup)
- Water (2 tbsp.)
- Sea salt (.5 tsp.)
- Raisins (1 cup)

Instructions:

1. Set the oven temperature at 350° Fahrenheit/177° Celsius.
2. Cover a cookie tray using a sheet of parchment baking paper.
3. Mix the spelt meal flour, dates, and sea salt using a food processor until thoroughly incorporated.
4. Pour it into a bowl and mix with the rest of the fixings.

5. Roll spoonfuls of cookie dough into a ball. Place them onto the baking tray and flatten with fingers or fork.
6. Bake for 18-25 minutes.
7. Wait for them to cool and enjoy!

Banana Nut Muffins

Total Time Required: 45 minutes
Yields Provided: 12

Ingredients Needed:
- Approved-flour (1.5 cups)
- Date sugar (.75 cup)
- Sea salt (.5 tsp.)
- Ripe burro bananas (2 medium)
- Walnut milk - homemade (.75 cup)
- Grapeseed oil (.25 cup)
- Ripe burro banana (1 medium)
- Key lime juice (1 tbsp.)
- Walnuts - chopped (.5 cup + more to sprinkle)
- Also Needed: 12-count muffin tin

Instructions:

1. Warm the oven to reach 400° Fahrenheit/204° Celsius.
2. Lightly grease the muffin pan cups or use liners.
3. Whisk each of the dry fixings in a big mixing container.
4. In a medium bowl, mash the banana and add with all of the wet fixings.

5. Combine the wet into dry, and stir until it's just starting to come together; don't over mix.
6. Mix in the walnuts and banana.
7. Portion the batter into the cups. Finish by sprinkling extra walnuts on top to your liking.
8. Bake until the muffins have risen and are golden brown on the edges (20-25 min.).
9. Cool them for about ten minutes before enjoying them.

Banoffee Crumble Pudding

Total Time Required: up to overnight
Yields Provided: 4

Ingredients Needed:
- Dried banana chips (3.5 oz./100g)
- Walnuts (2.5 oz./75 g)
- Coconut oil (1 tsp.)
- Squash
- Burro bananas (3)
- Springwater (6 fl oz./175m)
- Dates (6-10)
- Avocado (¼ of 1)
- Needed: Drinking glasses/ramekins (4)

Instructions:

1. *The Base*: Put 1/3 of the walnuts with the banana chips into a food processor.
2. Mix until it reaches a breadcrumb texture. Mix in the coconut oil and blend again.
3. Set aside two tablespoons of the mixture to decorate the dish later.
4. Scoop the rest between four dishes and pop it in the fridge to chill.
5. The Fruit Layer: Cut the squash into small pieces and cook in water until tender (15 min.).

6. Put the bananas, cooked squash, and water (25 ml/1 fl oz.) in a blender, mixing until smooth.
7. Add the dates (2-4) to sweeten (as desired).
8. Spoon over the cooled base and pop it back into the fridge.
9. *The Coating*: Soak the rest of the walnuts and six dates in cold spring water (3.5 fl oz./100ml) overnight or in hot water for two hours.
10. Put the walnuts, dates, and the soaking water with the avocado into the blender.
11. Use the high setting until it's a light - creamy texture.
12. Add more dates to increase toffee-like sweetness.
13. Spread the creamy mix over the refrigerated puddings.
14. Sprinkle the saved crumble mix over the tops.
15. Chill for at least an hour before serving.

<u>Berry Sorbet</u>

Total Time Required: 20 minutes + chill time (4 hours)
Yields Provided: 4

Ingredients Needed:
- Date sugar (.5 cup)
- Spelt flour (1.5 tsp.)
- Pureed strawberries (2 cups)
- Water (2 cups)

Instructions:

1. Dissolve the date sugar and flour in the water in a large saucepan using the low-temperature setting.
2. Boil until it's thickened, like syrup (10 min.). Transfer the pan from the burner and cool.
3. When the syrup is completely cooled, add the pureed fruit, and mix well.
4. Cut the sorbet into chunks, and process in a food processor until it's creamy.
5. Place in a plastic container and freeze uncovered until it is solid.
6. Put the sorbet back into the freezer and freeze it for another four hours.

Delicious Mango Cheesecake

Total Time Required: varies
Yields Provided: 8-12

Ingredients Needed:
The Crust:
- Walnuts (1 cup)
- Shredded desiccated soft-jelly coconut (.25 cup)
- Dates (1 cup)

The Filling:
- Soaked walnuts (2 cups)
- Homemade soft-jelly coconut milk (1 cup)
- Agave (.33 cup)
- Juice of 1 key lime
- Key lime zest (1 tbsp.)
- Mangos (2 large)
- Coconut oil (6 tbsp.)
- Also Needed 8x8 inch baking sheet with parchment paper

Instructions:

1. It's important to soak the walnuts in water overnight. Dump them in a colander to drain.
2. Peel and cut the mango into cubes.
3. Prepare the baking tray and set it aside.

4. Use a food processor/high-speed blender to mix the walnuts, dates, and shredded soft-jelly coconut until combined. Add a few dates if your dough is not sticky enough.
5. Push the dough into the bottom of your pan (as evenly as possible).
6. Pop the pan into the freezer.
7. In a food processor or high-speed blender, add the milk and nuts. Pulse them until thoroughly smooth (2-3 min.).
8. Add the coconut oil, agave syrup, key lime juice and zest, and mango cubes. Blend the fixings til it's thoroughly incorporated.
9. Scoop the "cheesecake mixture to the prepared pan, spreading evenly.
10. Pop in the freezer to firm up two to four hours before serving.
11. Serve frozen or thaw for a softer texture (10-15 min.).

Fall Apple Crumble

Total Time Required: 50-55 minutes
Yields Provided: 4

Ingredients Needed:
  The Filling:
  - Organic Braeburn apples (5)
  - Fresh spring water (2 tbsp.)
  - Ground cloves (.25 tsp.)
  - Sea salt (1 pinch)
  - Date sugar (1 tbsp.)
  The Topping:
  - Ground walnuts (.5 cup)
  - Spelt flour (.33 cup)
  - Amaranth flour (.33 cup)
  - Sea salt (.25 tsp. - heaping)
  - Crushed walnuts (.33 cup)
  - Date sugar (.33 cup)
  - Grapeseed oil (.33 cup)
  - Spring water (1 tsp./as needed)

Instructions:

1. Set the oven setting to reach 400°
   Fahrenheit/204° Celsius.
2. Lightly grease an 8x8-inch baking dish.

3. Peel and slice the apples into one-inch chunks.
4. Mix the apples with water in a saucepan. Simmer them using the low-temperature setting with a lid on the pan, stirring occasionally for 15 minutes.
5. Uncover, stir, and add the date sugar, ground cloves, and sea salt. The apples should be tender.
6. Prepare the topping in a food processor. Measure and add the flour, walnuts, date sugar, grapeseed oil, and sea salt, and pulse until crumbly. Add the water if needed.
7. Scoop the apple filling into the baking dish and sprinkle with the topping.
8. Bake until lightly crisp on top (18- 22 min.).

Fat-Free Peach Muffins

Total Time Required: 35-40 minutes
Yields Provided: 12 - may vary

Ingredients Needed:
- Agave syrup (1 tbsp.)
- Peaches (2 large/2 cups)
- Mashed burro banana (1.5 tsp.)
- Warm spring water (2 tbsp.)
- Key lime juice (2 tsp.)
- Homemade walnut milk (1.25 cups)
- Spelt flour (2 cups)
- Salt (.25 tsp.)
- Date sugar (.5 cup)
- Chopped walnuts (2 tbsp.)

Instructions:

1. Set the oven temperature setting to 400° Fahrenheit/204° Celsius.
2. Prepare the muffin pan by oiling it with a spritz of grapeseed oil.
3. Peel the peaches. If they are not ripe, dip them in boiling water for ½ minute and cool before peeling. Discard the pit. Chop into ½-inch pieces. Mix with agave syrup and place to the side for now.

4. Mix the lime juice and milk to the mashed burro banana. Mix thoroughly.
5. Whisk the sea salt, flour, and date sugar in a large mixing container.
6. Mix in the liquid components and stir just until combined. The batter should be thick.
7. Fold in the peaches, making sure they're evenly distributed throughout the batter.
8. Fill each cup to within ½-inch of the top. Use a knife to level the tops of each muffin and sprinkle with chopped walnuts.
9. Bake until a toothpick comes out clean (15-20 min.).
10. Wait for the muffins to cool before serving.

Sea Moss Panna Cotta

Total Time Required: 2.5 hours - varies
Yields Provided: 6

Ingredients Needed:
- Walnuts (2/3 cup)
- Soft-jelly coconut water (2 cups + 2 tbsp.)
- Bromide Plus Powder (1 tbsp.)
- Soft-jelly young coconut meat (.5 of 1 heaping cup)
- Agave syrup (.25 cup)
- Unrefined sea salt (1 pinch)
- Coconut oil (.25 cup + 1 tbsp.)
  Also Needed:
- Ramekins, molds, or espresso cups
- Nutribullet or similar high-speed blender

Instructions:

1. Soak the walnuts overnight.
2. Prepare by blending the walnuts and soft-jelly coconut water using the med-high speed setting until it's creamy smooth.
3. Scoop and strain the mixture through a nut milk bag or line a strainer using a double layer of cheesecloth and pour the mix

through. Squeeze out as much liquid as possible.

4. Use the blender and add the walnut milk, BromidePowder, coconut meat, and agave syrup.
5. Blend it using the medium-speed setting. Increase to the high-speed setting until thoroughly smooth (1-2 min.).
6. Grease the insides of the chosen cups with coconut oil (no need to grease cups/ramekins).
7. Scoop the mixture to fill the cups. Chill your sea moss panna cotta in the fridge until set and firm (2 hrs. minimum).
8. Add strawberries and agave syrup before serving.

Chapter 8
<u>Dr. Sebi's Beverages</u>

<u>Alkaline Electric Limeade</u>
Total Time Required: 4-5 minutes
Yields Provided: 2.5-3 cups

Ingredients Needed:
- Strawberries
- Regular or key limes
- Spring water
- Blue agave
- Ice
- Blender
⇊

Alkaline Limeade

Ingredients Needed:
- Spring water (2 cups)
- Lime juice (.25 cup)
- Agave (.25 cup)

Instructions:

1. Pour each of the fixings into a blender.
2. Blend it for ten seconds.
3. Pop it into the fridge to keep it chilled or serve it with a few ice cubes.

Alkaline Frozen Strawberry Limeade

Ingredients Needed:

- Lime juice (.25 cup)
- Strawberries (.5 cup)
- Spring water (1 cup)
- Agave (.25 cup)
- Ice Cubes (6-8)

Instructions:

1. Discard the leaves from the berries, and slice them into halves.
2. Toss each of the fixings into a blender.
3. Pulse it for ten seconds or until it's quietly mixing.

Kidney Cleanse Juice

Total Time Required: 8-10 minutes
Yields Provided: 1-2

Ingredients Needed:
- Soft-jelly coconut water (1-2 cups)
- Seeded cucumbers (4)
- Key limes (2-3)
- Basil or sweet basil leaves (1 bunch)
- Bromide Plus Powder (.5 tsp.)

Instructions:

1. Juice cucumbers, basil, and key limes. You can also process them in a high-speed blender with coconut water.
2. Serve the juice in a tall glass. Add coconut water and Bromide Powder.
3. Mix well and serve.

Sleepy-Time Drink

Total Time Required: 10 minutes
Yields Provided: 1-2

Ingredients Needed:
- Cooked quinoa (.25 cup)
- Amaranth greens (2 cups)
  Herbal Teas:
- Stomach Relief - Dr. Sebi's (.5 cup)
- Nerve/Stress Relief -Dr. Sebi's (.5 cup)
- Burro banana (1)
- Cherries (.25 cup)
- Agave syrup (as desired)

Instructions:

1. To prepare Dr. Sebi's Sleepy Time drink, start by brewing the tea according to instructions.
2. Let cool.
3. Blend all the fixings in a blender (high-speed is best) and enjoy!

Dr. Sebi's Infused Water Specialties

Use the following recipes to enjoy a refreshing drink.

For All Infused Water Recipes
- Water (5 cups water)
- Optional: Ice cubes (1 cup)

For Honeydew Melon & Seeded Cucumber
- Honeydew melon cubes (.5 cup)
- Seeded cucumber (1 thinly sliced)

For Strawberry - Basil & Key Lime
- Strawberries - stemmed & sliced (.5 cup)
- Fresh basil - leaves torn (5 large)
- Key lime (1 thinly sliced)

Apple Spice
- Organic apple (1 sliced)
- Cloves (1 tbsp.)

Blackberries & Seville Orange
- Blackberries (.5 pint)
- Seville orange (1 thinly sliced)

Watermelon Refresher

Total Time Required: 5-6 minutes
Yields Provided: 4

Ingredients Needed:
- Cubed watermelon (4 cups)
- Soft-jelly coconut water (2 cups)
- Date sugar (to your liking)
- Zest and juice (1 key lime)

Instructions:

1. Cube and add the watermelon, key lime juice, and zest into a food processor. Mix until it's creamy smooth.
2. Sweeten the mixture with the date sugar.
3. Serve in a tall glass.
4. Combine 2/3 watermelon mixture and 1/3 soft-jelly coconut water.
5. Mix with a spoon, and serve.

Conclusion

I hope you have enjoyed each of the new recipes in *Dr Sebi Smoothie*. I hope it was informative and provided you with all of the tools you need to achieve your goals - whatever they may be.

The next step is to decide what you would like to try first. Will it be one of Dr. Sebi's recipes for a smoothie? There is so much to choose from with this cookbook.

The creation of alkaline blood happens due to the scientific concept that the food you eat leaves behind a residue in the body. You can control this residue by controlling the foods you eat. Eating alkaline foods leads to alkaline blood. The traditional American diet includes great amounts of acidic food, which leads to acidic blood, and thus, disease.

This effect happens as a result of your body's metabolism. Metabolism is a large term that describes the breakdown of one thing to create energy for your body. It is all of the body's processes that work together to maintain a person's life in more specific terms. This process happens when you eat food, and it is broken down to create energy for your body to function. This process also happens on a smaller level in each cell as its cell components are broken down to create energy. When you eat food, your body's metabolism begins to act, and it breaks down the food to make energy. The creation of energy leads to something called *ash*, which is a by-product. This ash can be acidic or alkaline. The goal of this diet is to eliminate acidic ash and create only alkaline ash.

Finally, if you found this book useful in any way, a review on Amazon is always appreciated!